Essentials of Bedside Cardiology

CONTEMPORARY CARDIOLOGY

CHRISTOPHER P. CANNON, MD
SERIES EDITOR

Aging, Heart Disease and Its Management: Facts and Controversies, edited by
Niloo M. Edwards, MD, Mathew S. Maurer, MD, and Rachel B. Wellner, MD,
2003

Peripheral Arterial Disease: Diagnosis and Treatment, edited by *Jay D.*
Coffman, MD, and Robert T. Eberhardt, MD, 2003

Essentials of Bedside Cardiology: With a Complete Course in Heart Sounds and
Murmurs on CD, Second Edition, by *Jules Constant, MD, 2003*

Primary Angioplasty in Acute Myocardial Infarction, edited by *James E. Tcheng,*
MD, 2002

Cardiogenic Shock: Diagnosis and Treatment, edited by *David Hasdai, MD, Peter*
B. Berger, MD, Alexander Battler, MD, and David R. Holmes, Jr., MD, 2002

Management of Cardiac Arrhythmias, edited by *Leonard I. Ganz, MD, 2002*

Diabetes and Cardiovascular Disease, edited by *Michael T. Johnstone and Aristidis*
Veves, MD, DSC, 2001

Blood Pressure Monitoring in Cardiovascular Medicine and Therapeutics,
edited by *William B. White, MD, 2001*

Vascular Disease and Injury: Preclinical Research, edited by *Daniel I. Simon, MD,*
and Campbell Rogers, MD 2001

Preventive Cardiology: Strategies for the Prevention and Treatment of Coronary
Artery Disease, edited by *JoAnne Micale Foody, MD, 2001*

Nitric Oxide and the Cardiovascular System, edited by *Joseph Loscalzo, MD,*
PhD and Joseph A. Vita, MD, 2000

Annotated Atlas of Electrocardiography: A Guide to Confident
Interpretation, by *Thomas M. Blake, MD, 1999*

Platelet Glycoprotein IIb/IIIa Inhibitors in Cardiovascular Disease,
edited by *A. Michael Lincoff, MD, and Eric J. Topol, MD, 1999*

Minimally Invasive Cardiac Surgery, edited by *Mehmet C. Oz, MD and Daniel*
J. Goldstein, MD, 1999

Management of Acute Coronary Syndromes, edited by *Christopher P. Cannon, MD,*
1999

Essentials of Bedside Cardiology

WITH

A Complete Course
in Heart Sounds and Murmurs on CD

SECOND EDITION

Jules Constant, MD, FACC

Clinical Associate Professor of Medicine
State University of New York at Buffalo School of Medicine
Buffalo, NY

Humana Press ✳ Totowa, New Jersey

ANSI Z39.48-1984 (American National Standards Institute) Permanence of Paper for Printed Library Materials.

Cover design by Patricia F. Cleary.

Printed in the United States of America.   10 9 8 7 6 5 4 3 2 1

Library of Congress Cataloging in Publication Data

Constant, Jules, 1922-
   Essentials of bedside cardiology : with a complete course in heart sounds and murmurs on CD / by Jules Constant.--2nd ed.
      p. ; cm. -- (Contemporary cardiology)
   Rev. ed. of: Essentials of bedside cardiology for students and house staff. 1st ed. c1989.
   Includes bibliographical references and index.
   ISBN 1-58829-142-1 (alk. paper)
      1. Heart--Examination. 2. Heart--Diseases--Diagnosis. 3. Heart--Sounds. 4. Medical history taking. I. Constant, Jules, 1922- Essentials of bedside cardiology for students and house staff. II. Title. III. Contemporary cardiology (Totowa, N.J. : Unnumbered)
      [DNLM: 1. Heart Diseases--diagnosis. 2. Heart Sounds. 3. Physical Examination. WG 141 C757ea 2002]
   RC683.C593 2002
   616.1'2--dc21

                                                                                          2002190222

To Elizabeth, my wife, without whom this book might never have been published

Preface

Essentials of Bedside Cardiology, Second Edition, like the first edition, is designed for those who wish to balance technological advances with increased personal skill in history taking and physical examination.

It is important to teach physicians that all technologies now in use for diagnosing cardiovascular disorders, such as echocardiography, can have false positive and false negative results. It is not always wise to rely on these technologies alone; indeed, they may not even be available in some settings. Even when the full panoply of up-to-date techniques is at the physician's disposal, the patient may not be a good candidate for an echocardiogram, or the technician or reader may not be well qualified, or the equipment itself may be substandard. Technology must be combined with physical examination to decide what is true and what is false.

The practice of expert history taking and physical examination returns the physician to the actual patient, where the physician can feel like a "real doctor" rather than a mere interpreter of laboratory data.

Essentials of Bedside Cardiology, Second Edition, strives to teach and not simply to tell the facts, relying on three basic methods derived from the psychology of teaching and learning:

1. Explain the facts.
2. Use a question and answer format—the Socratic method.
3. Provide tricks or mnemonics to help the reader remember the facts.

The value of the Socratic method is its ability to focus attention and stimulate thinking. The format of *Essentials of Bedside Cardiology, Second Edition,* supports this goal by allowing the reader to cover up the answer and so use the book as a programmed learning tool.

A demonstration of all the heart sounds and murmurs with detailed explanations of what is being heard is provided on the enclosed CD. No simulators have been used. In addition, the use of phonocardiograms and pulse tracings for teaching is encouraged throughout the text.

The index also is a learning tool, having been compiled by me, based on 40 years of teaching experience, with the goal of efficiently guiding the reader to the information needed. The glossary, too, is designed for all levels of readers, constituting a virtual encyclopedia of terms for the cardiologist, student, and noncardiologist alike. Terms that are fully explained in the glossary are typeset in boldface throughout the text as one more pedagogical aid.

Essentials of Bedside Cardiology, Second Edition, is the only book that teaches how to recognize normal jugular waves using updated terminology, how to measure jugular pressure accurately, how to record auscultation findings with an auscultogram, how to tell cardiac function by the blood pressure cuff and Valsalva method, how to diagnose cardiomegaly on an X-ray without using the outdated cardiothoracic ratio, and how to tell whether the apex beat is due to the right or left ventricle. It also gives the latest explanation for the changing loudness of the first heart sound with changing P–R intervals and updates methods for recording and taking an accurate blood pressure.

Jules Constant, MD, FACC

Contents

1 The Checklist in History Taking

ADVANTAGES OF A CHECKLIST

Traditionally, students have learned to take a history by memorizing a standard checklist and have been warned that a checklist should not be used in front of the patient.

When the opinions of patients were solicited concerning the reading of questions in front of them, it was found that patients either did not recall that the physician had been reading the questions, or if the patient had been to other doctors, they would often claim that it was the first time they had a thorough history taken.

Some of the advantages of reading an organized list of questions are:

1. The final history as written on paper may be very short because no negative findings need be recorded; otherwise it is necessary to list all negative findings for the reader to know what has been asked.

2. The history can be taken more rapidly with a list of questions than without, because you are not trying to recall your place as would be necessary with a memorized checklist, especially if the patient rambles.

3. Upon leaving the patient, there is no feeling of insecurity due to fear that you may have forgotten to ask something.

Cardiological diagnosis can be learned from the checklist in this chapter. An asterisk before each important symptom refers the physician to another page that lists further questions suggesting a differential diagnosis. In this way, physicians can take a good chief complaint history, and they also learn the differential diagnosis of all important symptoms.

The checklist proposed here is not to be used as a "check-off" list with yes or no answers but rather as a "reminder" list. The patient's answers to the reminder list can be taken down in an unorganized form on separate sheets and later reorganized under a few headings, such as:

1. Chief complaint (why patient came or was referred, and who referred). How long before seeing you or before admission?

2. History of chief complaint or complaints. For example, if the patient has chest pain, write the complete story of the chest pain from the follow-up questions of the checklist.

3. Other etiologies pertinent to the chief complaint. These headings should contain the word "Possibilities"; for example, if the patient has known valvular disease, "Rheumatic Heart Disease Possibilities" would be an appropriate heading.

REMINDER LIST HISTORY

If the patient has had cardiac surgery, indicate the date, place, type of operation, name of surgeon. Were cardiac symptoms alleviated? Catheterization results? Were there surgical complications, e.g., emboli or infections? Treatment after surgery, e.g., anticoagulants?

Left Ventricular Failure or High Left Atrial Pressure Possibilities

Note: An asterisk before a question indicates that if the patient answers yes to that question, you should turn to a later page that gives the differential diagnosis of that symptom by means of more questions.

*1. Dyspnea, cough, or wheeze on exertion, on hills or on stairs? (If yes, see p. 7.)

*2. Orthopnea? (If yes, see p. 8.)

*3. Paroxysmal nocturnal dyspnea? (If yes, see p. 9.)

4. Heart failure symptoms in pregnancy? (If in first trimester, may be due to placental product.)

5. Therapy with low-salt diet or drugs? (Indicate dose and if helped.) Why stopped? Side effects? If digitalis, did patient have gastrointestinal symptoms, weakness [1], faintness, dizziness, visual disturbances, or palpitations? If diuretics (loop or thiazide?), were there muscle cramps or weakness? Preload or afterload reducers used? Drugs used that could precipitate borderline failure, e.g., beta blockers, calcium blockers, or disopyramide?

Peripheral Venous Congestion or Pseudo Right Heart Failure Possibilities

*1. Peripheral edema, maximum and minimum weight? (If yes, see p. 9.)

2. Abdominal swelling? (If before orthopnea, consider tamponade. (See p. 5 for tamponade symptoms.) Right upper abdominal pain with exercise or bending discomfort? (Suggests hepatomegaly.)

Low Output State Possibilities

1. Weakness or fatigue? Afternoon nap necessary? When last able to do normal activities comfortably? Most strenuous activity in past few months?

2. Cold extremities? How long?

3. Excess perspiration? (A sign of failure in infants.) With warm hands, suggests hyperthyroidism; with cold hands, suggests neurocirculatory asthenia (psychoneurosis) or failure.

4. Insomnia? (May indicate **Cheyne-Stokes respiration** with hyperpnea on dozing.)

5. Nocturia with polyuria? (May be daytime failure compensating at rest.)

6. Orthostatic faintness.

Fixed Output State Possibilities

*1. Syncope, presyncope, or dizziness? (If yes, see p. 7.)

*2. Chest pain or tightness? (If yes, see p. 11.)

Chamber Enlargement Possibilities

1. Trepopnea? (Cannot lie horizontally in bed, but not due to heart failure.)

*2. Palpitations or awareness of heart beat? (If yes, see p. 13.)

3. Told of enlarged heart? (From ECG, X-ray, echocardiogram, or physical examination?) Date of last chest X-ray (portable?), echocardiogram, and ECG?

ETIOLOGIES ───────────────────────────────

Rheumatic Heart Disease Possibilities

1. History of rheumatic fever with joint pains or chorea (twitches or clumsiness for a few months)? Red, swollen joints, or only fever plus murmur as a child? Therapy with prophylactic penicillin? Family history of rheumatic fever? Murmur history (for school examination, operation, insurance, or military service)? Was it the result of cardiac catheterization or an echocardiogram? When and where done? Were there "growing pains" or nocturnal leg pains (not rheumatic)?

Complications of Rheumatic Heart Disease

1. If mitral stenosis; hemoptysis, hoarseness, Ortner syndrome, or cardiovocal syndrome. (pressure of large left atrium on large pulmonary artery against recurrent laryngeal nerve), or embolic phenomena (hematuria, pleurisy, unilateral weakness, or partial vision loss in one eye due to calcium emboli from aortic valve)?

2. If aortic stenosis: exertional dyspnea, syncope, or angina (classic aortic stenosis triad)?

Boldface type indicates that the term is explained in the glossary.

3. If aortic regurgitation: nocturnal angina or awareness of large pulsations in arms, neck, or chest?

4. If **infective endocarditis**: severe night sweats, dental work, or embolic phenomena, such as back pain or cerebrovascular accident?

Ischemic Heart Disease *Possibilities*

*1. Chest pain, tightness, or pressure? (If yes, see p. 11.)

2. Previous myocardial infarction? Symptoms and hospital course? Postinfarction drugs, such as beta blockers and aspirin, used?

3. Risk factors:

   a. Major: hypertension, high cholesterol or triglycerides, low HDL, smoking, family history of infarction at early age?

   b. Minor: diabetes, premature menopause, intermittent claudication, gout, high uric acid [2]? Is patient type A (slightly hostile, aggressive, and impatient)? Stressful job or home life? On diet or taking drugs to decrease lipids?

   c. Marked postprandial somnolence (suggests severe hypertriglyceridemia, or insulin resistance.)

Hypertensive Heart Disease Possibilities

*1. Hypertension? (If yes, see p. 14.)

High Output Failure Possibilities

1. Anemia: under treatment? Heavy periods, bleeding piles or melena? Upper gastrointestinal surgery (B_{12} deficiency)? Sickle cell disease history? Lead contact? Radiation or anticancer drugs?

2. Thyrotoxicosis: heat intolerance, warm skin, weight loss, polydipsia, polyuria, excess perspiration, frequent stools, restlessness, muscle weakness on climbing, or palpitations?

3. **Beriberi**: evidence of alcoholism with a poor diet? Bartender job? Fad diets or peripheral neuritis? Long time on large-dose diuretics?

Cor Pulmonale Possibilities

1. Chronic obstructive pulmonary disease: smokes? Easier to breathe leaning forward? Were pulmonary function tests performed? Told of emphysema or experienced chronic cough with wheezing and sputum? Coal miner? Abnormal chest X-ray? Marked obesity? Pickwickian syndrome.

2. Asthma: is wheezing helped by bronchodilators? Seasonal dyspnea?

3. Pulmonary emboli: is there is a history of phlebitis or oral contraceptives? Sudden dyspnea at rest with pleurisy or faintness with cold sweat or hemoptysis? Recently on long auto or airline trip or had trauma or surgery?

4. Primary pulmonary hypertension: **Raynaud's phenomenon** [3] or fixed output symptoms?

Pericarditis, Effusion, Constriction, or Tamponade Possibilities

Etiologies

Chest trauma: postcardiotomy or postmyocardial infarction syndrome (Dressier's syndrome) with fever, pleurisy, and polyserositis, as long as 2 months after surgery. Chest radiation, uremia, metastatic carcinoma, lymphoma, leukemia, lupus, rheumatoid arthritis, tuberculosis contact, or recent viremia. Drugs: procainamide, hydralazine, or isoniazid.

Symptoms of Pericarditis

1. Chest pain on motion, swallowing, or inspiration.

2. Past history of pericarditis (idiopathic type may be recurrent).

3. Epigastric pain for a few days before chest pain.

Symptoms of Tamponade

1. Dyspnea on exertion, especially if it stops immediately on stopping exertion.

2. Edema or abdominal swelling beginning before or simultaneously with dyspnea on exertion is highly suggestive of **tamponade.**

Myocarditis, Endocarditis, and Other Heart Disease Possibilities

1. Recent influenza-like illness with myalgia?

2. **Infective endocarditis**: drug addiction, fevers, surgical or dental procedures, or recent back pain?

3. Collagen disease: Raynaud's phenomenon, dysphagia, arthritis, or arthralgia?

4. Ankylosing spondylitis: hip, sciatic, or back pain, especially on awakening or increasing with coughing?

5. Hypophosphatemia: high intake of phosphorus-binding antacids, e.g., aluminum hydroxide? Acute alcohol excess?

6. Hypertrophic cardiomyopathies: sudden death in family? Angina or syncope after exercise? Dyspnea not helped by digitalis?

7. Luetic aortic regurgitation or aneurysm: veneral disease or hoarseness (aneurysm compressing recurrent laryngeal nerve)?

Infiltrative Cardiomyopathies

1. Hemochromatosis: diabetic? Skin color changes? Liver failure: impotence, upper abdominal pain, gynecomastia, or arthritis? Frequent transfusions?
2. Sarcoidosis: syncope (from atrioventricular [AV] block), chest X-ray abnormality, kidney stones, or eye symptoms (uveitis)?
3. Amyloidosis: postural hypotension, peripheral neuropathy, or skin lesions, especially if pruritic or bleed when scratched? Angina? Weakness? Dysarthria? Purpura?
4. Parasitic disease: trichinosis or Chagas' disease (eaten rare meat or been in foreign country)?
5. Hypothyroidism or myxedema. See follow-up questions 4 under hormonal causes. See under Peripheral edema, hormonal causes, p. 9.

Cardiac Tumors

1. **Atrial myxoma**: embolic phenomena, fevers, arthralgias, skin lesions, paresthesias, presyncope or syncope with changes of posture?
2. **Carcinoid**: diarrhea, wheezing, or flushing of face, neck, and front of chest for minutes or days?

Congenital Heart Disease Possibilities

To Be Asked Only if Patient Is an Infant

1. Frequent pneumonias (suggests increased lung blood flow)?
2. Excess perspiration (sign of failure in infants)?
3. Mother aware of infant's heartbeat or vibration or thrill?

To Be Asked if Patient Is an Infant, Child, or Adult

1. Murmur at birth? (Suggests stenotic lesion. If delayed a few weeks, suggests left-to-right shunt).
2. Results of cardiac catheterization.
3. Pregnancy with rubella? (Suggests **persistent ductus, ventricular septal defect, atrial septal defect**, stenosis, pulmonary arterial [not valvular] stenosis, or **tetralogy of Fallot**.)
4. Normal growth and development? (High birth weight suggests transposition.)

5. The mother's pregnancy: If viral illness, may produce myocarditis in newborn. If diabetes, suggests transposition. Age of mother when pregnant? (If in 40s, suggests tetralogy of Fallot.)

6. Family history of congenital heart disease or murmur?

7. Cyanosis? From birth, suggests **transposition** or tetralogy. If delayed until teens or middle age, suggests **Eisenmenger's syndrome** or **Ebstein's anomaly**. If with crying, feeding, or warm bath, or if only with syncope, suggests tetralogy. If differential cyanosis and clubbing (fingers pink but toes blue), suggests ductus with Eisenmenger's syndrome. Frequent phlebotomies?

8. Stroke? (Consider embolus from endocardial fibroelastosis, idiopathic cardiomyopathy, or paradoxical embolus from right atrium. If cyanotic, consider cerebral abscess.)

9. Crying during feeding: suggests angina due to anomalous left coronary artery.

To Be Asked Only if Patient Is a Child or Adult

1. Hoarseness? (Suggests large ductus or **primary pulmonary hypertension**.)

2. Mental retardation? (Consider the Down syndrome or supravalvular aortic stenosis.)

3. Hypertrophic osteoarthropathy with swelling, pain, warmth, and lower extremity tenderness? (Consider ductus with Eisenmenger's syndrome.)

4. Recurrent bleeding from nose, lips, and mouth with melena and hemoptysis due to hereditary hemorrhagic telangiectasia or Rendu-Osler-Weber disease? (Suggests pulmonary AV fistula, especially if cyanotic.)

5. Presyncope or syncope? If on exertion, suggests aortic stenosis or primary pulmonary hypertension; if with straining or after sleep and with cyanosis, suggests tetralogy. If at rest, consider epilepsy or complete **atrioventricular block** with **Stokes-Adams attack**.

6. Squatting? (Suggests tetralogy, pulmonary atresia, or Eisenmenger's syndrome.)

7. Headaches, epistaxis, leg fatigue, cold legs, or claudication? (Suggests **coarctation**.)

FOLLOW-UP QUESTIONS ────────────────────

1. If Patient Says Yes to Dyspnea on Exertion

Orientation

When was the patient last able to do normal activities comfortably? How far can the patient walk on the level or stairs before dyspnea? Is walking rate slower? Can patient walk and talk simultaneously? The most strenuous activity performed in the past few months?

Etiologies

1. Failure: effect of digitalis, diuretics, low salt intake, or afterload treatment? Is there orthopnea, paroxysmal nocturnal dyspnea, or cough and wheeze on exertion? (If suddenly worse, suggests ruptured chordae, atrial fibrillation, pulmonary embolus, or acute infarction). If on digitalis, any gastrointestinal or visual symptoms? Weakness, faintness, dizziness, or palpitations?

2. Anginal equivalent: (One-third of patients with angina have simultaneous dyspnea without heart failure.) Lasts 10–20 min? With nausea, perspiration, or occasionally with angina? Had Holter monitor?

3. Arrhythmia: with abnormal rhythm or palpitations? Begins and ends suddenly? Ever checked pulse when short of breath?

4. Anxiety: nervous breakdown, or tranquilizer history, or hyperventilated with paresthesias, cold perspiration, palpitations, and days without dyspnea? (Suggests **neurocirculatory asthenia**.)

5. Pulmonary dysfunction: associated with weight gain? Asthma: wheezes helped by bronchodilators? Evidence of emphysema, smokes, coughs with sputum? Pulmonary function results? Pulmonary embolism: sudden shortness of breath, syncope with hemoptysis, chest pains, cold sweats, phlebitis, or varicose veins? Is patient pregnant or on contraceptive pills? Recent long trip? Pneumothorax: sudden shortness of breath or inspiratory chest or shoulder pain with dry cough?

6. Severe anemia: has patient had bleeding ulcers, hemorrhoids, or excessive bleeding from the uterus; melena; sickle cell disease; gastrectomy? Been treated with vitamin B_{12} or iron? Pins-and-needles sensation?

7. Compression of pulmonary artery or bronchus: results of last chest X-ray?

2. If Patient Says Yes to Orthopnea

Orientation

When did it begin? Spontaneous, or told by physician to use more pillows?

Severity

How high must the head be? How soon after the patient lies down does it begin? (Orthopnea begins in less than a minute.)

Etiologies

1. Trepopnea: horizontal discomfort not due to heart failure, occasionally due to feeling large heart against bed when on left side, or due to musculoskeletal pain or dizziness, or to hypoxia from lying on side of lung with pneumonia or cancer.

2. Markedly decreased vital capacity: no complete relief at any chest elevation (as with severe mitral stenosis)? Relieved if the patient remains supine? (Suggests pulmonary hypertension.)

3. If Patient Says Yes to Paroxysmal Nocturnal Dyspnea (PND)

Orientation

When did PND begin? How frequently does it recur?

Due to LV Failure

a. How long after the patient is asleep does it occur? (Redistribution of fluid takes 2–4 h to raise left atrial pressure.)
b. Does the patient dangle legs to get relief? (If not, it is not PND.)
c. Duration? (It should take 10–30 min to redistribute fluid back into tissue.)
d. With cough, wheezing, or frothy, pink sputum?

Not Due to LV Failure

a. Occurs also during the day? (If so, then it is not PND.)
b. No effect of digitalis, diuretics, and afterload therapy?
c. Awakens with palpitations, chronic cough, postnasal drip, or nocturia before shortness of breath noted?
d. Awakens with chest pain or tightness? (Nocturnal angina.)

4. If Patient Says Yes to Peripheral Edema

Orientation

When did it begin? Shoes too tight? Does edema extend to the knees? Is it gone in the morning? Effect of digitalis, diuretics, and afterload treatment?

Etiologies

1. Cardiac: helped by cardiac-failure drugs?
2. Stasis or obstructive edema: began with weight gain or pregnancy? Tight panty girdle or varicose veins or phlebitis? Shirt collar tight and face swollen? (Suggests superior vena cave obstruction.) Abdominal swelling? (Suggests constriction, tamponade, or ovarian cancer.)
3. Hormonal causes: premenstrual syndrome; breast fullness, headache, and mood changes? On estrogens or contraceptive pills? Aldosteronism: hypertension, weakness, tetany, paresthesias, or a high licorice intake? Myxedema: voice

change, dry skin, cold intolerance, sluggishness, weight gain, constipation, menorrhagia, or decreased hearing? Thyroid tests?

4. Intermittent idiopathic edema of women: menstrual disorders?

5. Drug-induced: on vasodilators, nonsteroidal anti-inflammatory agents calcium blockers, or estrogens?

6. Renal: facial and hand edema? Worse in the morning?

7. Cirrhosis: alcoholism, hepatitis, or jaundice?

8. Constriction: Did edema begin before the dyspnea?

9. Severe COPD due to: (a) high intraabdominal pressure durinq expiration, as well as inspiration; (b) high CO_2 dilating afferent renal arterioles more than efferents.

5. If Patient Says Yes to Presyncope, Syncope, or Dizziness

Orientation

When did it begin? Duration and frequency? By dizziness does the patient mean faintness, loss of balance, lightheadedness, blurred vision, sinking feeling, floating sensation, unsteadiness, swaying, swimming, or vertigo?

Etiologies

1. Epilepsy: how long unconscious? Is mind clear after? Prodrume? Began with a twitch? Sore tongue, incontinence, or head trauma? Family history? Were convulsions witnessed? Ever had EEG or neurological examination? Were anticonvulsants administered?

2. Acute infarction: preceded or followed by chest or arm discomfort, shortness of breath, or perspiration?

3. Hysterical: always in the presence of someone else? Paresthesias or dyspnea also (hyperventilation)? Ever injured self?

4. Orthostatic: after prolonged bed rest? On antihypertensives or dialysis? Autonomic abnormalities: diabetes, nocturnal diarrhea, impotence, peripheral neuritis, or absent sweating? Worse if hot or fatigued? Large varicose veins?

5. Excess bleeding: piles, melena, menorrhagia, on anticoagulants, trauma? (A ruptured spleen may produce symptoms a week after trauma.)

6. Carotid insufficiency: unilateral blindness, weakness, paresthesias, dysarthria, or aphasia for a few minutes or hours?

7. Vasovagal: preceded by nausea or sinking epigastric feeling? Skin wet and pale after? Associated with tight collar, head turning, or hyperextension? (Suggests hypersensitive carotid sinus.)

8. Fixed output or obstruction to flow: known pulmonary hypertension or stenosis? Syncope after exercise cessation? (Suggests hypertrophic obstructive cardiomyopathy.) Atrial myxoma, fevers, embolic phenomena, or dyspnea with changes of posture?

9. **Stokes-Adams attacks**: flushed after the attack and slow pulse noted at the time?

10. Pulmonary embolism: preceded by lightheadedness with or without dyspnea and pleuritic pain, hemoptysis, or cold sweat? Long trip sitting?

11. Cough or micturition syncope?

12. "Drop attacks" (sudden loss of postural tone without losing consciousness): a deadweight when someone tried to raise body? (Pressure on soles of feet regains postural tone.)

13. Stroke: unilateral weakness or slurred speech?

14. Cardiac syncope: with palpitations? Long Q–T syndrome (precipitated by quinidine, disopyramide, exercise, fatigue, anxiety, or a sudden loud noise or preceded by nausea or headache)? Erythromycin-type drug?

15. Sick sinus syndrome: history of slow pulse or palpitations as in bradycardia-tachycardia syndrome?

16. Cyanotic heart disease, tetralogy of Fallot.

6. If Patient Says Yes to Chest Pain or Pressure

Orientation

When did it begin, and how often does it recur? Longest and shortest time between episodes?

1. Site: (Ask patient to show you. Do not ask patient to point. If classic angina, the fist or hand will be over sternum or across chest. If the patient points, it is likely nonanginal.) Is there radiation? Several chest pains? Classic angina radiates to medial side of forearm to thumb. May radiate to jaw, anywhere on abdomen, to surgical scar or interscapular area.

2. Character: classic angina with tightness and pressure? (Any kind of discomfort can be angina.)

3. Nonangina: points to site with one finger? Lasts less than 5 s or more than 30 min? Increases with inspiration, local pressure, or one movement of the arms or chest? Relieved immediately when patient lies down? Reaches maximum immediately?; (Suggests dissection.) Seeks relief by walking? Radiates to lateral forearm or thumb?

Etiologies

1. Coronary obstruction: classic angina precipitated mainly after first exertion in morning, by food or cold air and anything that increases heart rate or afterload. With pallor, flatulence, nausea, sweating, or dyspnea? Relieved by drugs that decrease preload, afterload, heart rate, or inotropism? Risk factors: diabetes, hypertension, artificial menopause, contraceptive use, smoking, gout, **intermittent claudication**, previous infarction, family history of coronary disease, increased cholesterol or low HDL?

2. Vasospastic angina (Prinzmetal's angina): at rest, especially at night toward morning? Precipitated by cold air? Good and bad days?

3. Unstable angina: occurs more frequently with less provocation, lasts longer, or at rest?

Noncoronary Causes

1. Pericarditis: worse supine and with inspiration? Relieved by leaning forward? Worse with leg elevation, swallowing, or extending neck. May be referred to left neck, shoulder, and arm by phrenic nerve. Also to abdomen, especially in children. Unlike angina, it is less likely to be retrosternal and more likely left-sided. It may be influenced by each heart beat.

2. Congenital absence of pericardium? Brought on by lying on the left side? Lasts a few seconds or minutes? Relieved by changing position in bed?

3. Esophagitis or spasm: burning pain on eating or lying down? Acid reflux (water brash)? Relieved by antacids or hot drinks? Hiatal hernia on X-ray? Dysphagia?

4. Root neuritis: had herpes zoster or chest injury? Radiates to radial side of the hand? (Suggests herniated cervical disk.) Cervical root compression syndrome: brought on by arm or head movements?

5. Scalenus anticus or thoracic outlet syndrome: paresthesias and pain along the ulnar distribution? Worse with head turning, abduction, lifting weight, working with hands over the shoulder, or sleeping on side?

6. Costochondritis, myositis, or local neuritis: brought on by local pressure?

7. Fixed output syndrome: known severe aortic or pulmonary stenosis or pulmonary hypertension?

8. Aortic dissection (pain similar to infarction. If in the back, the aneurysm is probably distal to subclavian): pain maximum at onset? Radiates to abdomen or legs? Pain tearing or ripping? Presyncope or syncope with pain? Does it begin in epigastrium and radiate to chest? Has Marfan syndrome or coarctation?

9. Acute infarction (the site either similar to the patient's chronic angina or lower but more widespread): with perspiration, faintness, syncope, nausea, or vomiting? May pace to try for relief.

   Note: Epigastric pain with radiation to the neck is almost always due to right coronary disease. Epigastric pain with no radiation means left circumflex disease. Cheat pain radiating down the right arm is usually due to inferior infarction.

10. Aortic stenosis: High velocity jet produces Venturi effect and reduces coronary flow.

    Note: The area of the normally open aortic valve is $3-4$ cm². Symptoms usually do not develop until the area is reduced to about a third of normal ($1-1\frac{1}{2}$ cm²). However, symptoms may not develop until the orifice is only 0.5 cm².

11. Pulmonary infarction with intercostal tenderness; increases with arm or chest movement.

7. If Patient Says Yes to Palpitations

Orientation

When did they begin? Shortest and longest duration, and length of time between episodes?

Types and Rates of Arrhythmias

1. Is beat continuous, or only occasional strong beat? Regular or irregular? (Ask patient to tap out rate and rhythm.) Ever taken own pulse during palpitations? Is ECG abnormal? (Consider **Wolff-Parkinson-White syndrome.**)

2. Ectopic tachycardia vs sinus tachycardia: does it begin and end suddenly? Occurs at rest or always with exertion? Any maneuvers tried to stop it?

Etiologies

1. Much tea, coffee, cola, or alcohol? On drugs such as digitalis, diuretics, anticholinergics, or cocaine?

2. Thyroid disease (heat intolerance, etc.; see under High Output Failure Possibilities in Checklist) or pheochromocytoma (flushing, headaches, or perspiration)?

3. Sick sinus syndrome with tachycardia-bradycardia: is there presyncope, syncope, or slow pulse?

8. If Patient Says Yes to Hypertension

Orientation

When was patient first told? If treated, for how long? Side effects?

Severity

Past blood pressure readings? Had convulsions, strokes, headaches (occipital morning headache suggests severe hypertension), nocturnal dyspnea or dyspnea on exertion, orthopnea, or epistaxis? X-rays and ECG abnormal?

Etiologies

1. Essential hypertension: family history? Onset date? (Essential hypertension usually begins in fourth decade.)
2. Renal: kidney infections or stones, back injury, urinary frequency, polyuria, prostatism, gout, or severe diabetes?
3. Coarctation: cold legs, claudication, or shoulder girdle pain?
4. Pheochromocytoma: flushing, pounding headaches, dizziness, perspiration, palpitations, nausea, chest pains, paresthesias, or weight loss?
5. Aldosteronism: episodic or continual weakness, tetany, polyuria (mostly nocturnal), or polydipsia?
6. Hormonal: on contraceptives? Cushing's syndrome: on steroids? Hirsutism, easy bruising, acne, weakness, kidney stones, emotional lability, or depression? Hyperparathyroidism: peptic ulcer (calcium stimulates gastric secretion), renal calculi, constipation, lethargy, or polyuria?

NEW YORK HEART ASSOCIATION FUNCTIONAL AND THERAPEUTIC CLASSIFICATION

This functional classification (4) refers to fatigue, dyspnea, or angina. The original classification is too long to memorize, and a simplified one follows.

Class 1: The patient is asymptomatic, or symptoms occur on extraordinary exertion. (There is no class 0, or classification for a patient with a normal heart.)

Class 2: Symptoms occur on ordinary exertion.

Class 3: Symptoms occur on less than ordinary exertion.

Class 4: Symptoms occur at rest or on slight exertion.

Note: The functional classification is easily remembered if one simply re-
members the words "ordinary exertion," because Class 1 simply adds
"extra" in front of ordinary, Class 2 adds no words in front of ordinary,
and Class 3 adds "less than" in front of ordinary.

REFERENCES

1. Lely, A. H., and vanEnter, C. H. Non-cardiac symptoms of digitalis intoxication. *Am. Heart J.* 83:149, 1972.
2. Fessel, W. J. High uric acid as an indicator of cardiovascular disease: Independence from obesity. *Am. J. Med.* 68:3, 1980.
3. Walcott, G., Burchell, H. B., and Brown, A. L., Jr. Primary pulmonary hypertension. *Am. J. Med.* 49:70, 1970.
4. Criteria Committee, New York Heart Association. *Diseases of the Heart and Blood Vessels: Nomencluture and Criteria for Diagnosis* (6th ed.). Boston: Little, Brown, 1964, p. 114.

2 Cardiac Clues from Physical Appearance

SKIN

1. What is meant by cyanosis?

    ANS: Cyanosis is the bluish or purplish color imparted to the skin and mucous membranes, usually the result of at least 5 mg per dL of reduced hemoglobin in the surface capillaries, but occasionally due to an abnormal hemoglobin such as sulfmethemoglobin.

2. How can you distinguish central from peripheral cyanosis clinically?

    ANS: Central cyanosis is seen in warm as well as cold areas (compare with the tongue of a normal patient). In African American patients, evidence of central cyanosis may be seen in the conjunctiva. Definite central cyanosis is not usually recognized unless the arterial oxygen saturation is lowered to about 80%. Peripheral cyanosis is seen only in cool areas such as the nail beds, nose, cheeks, earlobes, and the outer surface of lips, where slow flow decreases the amount of hemoglobin in the surface capillaries. If **clubbing** is present or if the hands are warm, the cyanosis is probably central.

The earliest sign of clubbing is probably the reduction or absence of the groove where the root of the nail slips under the skin. Moist, warm fingertips are often associated signs.

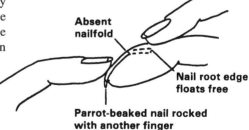

Absent nailfold

Nail root edge floats free

Parrot-beaked nail rocked with another finger

3. How should you test for mild clubbing?

    ANS: a. Look for obliteration of the normal angle between the base of the nail and the proximal skin.

Boldface type indicates that the term is explained in the glossary.

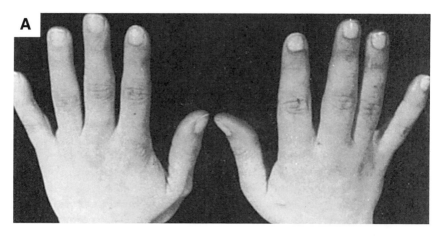

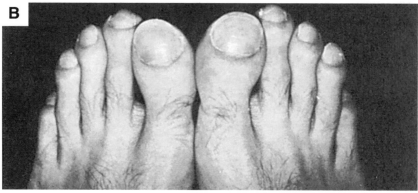

The feet of this 23-year-old man with a reversed shunt through a persistent ductus were cyanotic and clubbed, while his hands were normal.

       b. Approach the nail bed from behind and feel the edge of the nail root floating free when the distal portion of the nail is depressed with another finger.

4. What can cause clubbing, besides cyanotic heart disease?

    ANS.: Hypertrophic osteoarthropathy as in cancer of the lung, infective endocarditis, and severe ulcerative colitis.

       Note: Cancer of the lung is the most common cause of painful clubbing.

5. What is differential cyanosis and what is its significance?

    ANS: Differential cyanosis means that the fingers are pink but the toes are cyanotic (and usually clubbed). It signifies the presence of a persistent ductus arteriosus (PDA) with a reversed right-to-left shunt due to pulmonary hypertension (**Eisenmenger syndrome**). The left hand may also be cyanotic, because the ductus may be located at the branching part of the left subclavian artery.

6. What are the skin signs secondary to the small emboli of **infective endocarditis**?

   ANS: a. Clubbing.
         b. Splinter hemorrhages in the nails. (Most splinter hemorrhages are not embolic and are due to repeated jarring. Since they are in the nail substance, they move with the nail as it grows and they extend to the distal nail edge. Embolic splinters are subungual and usually do not extend to the distal nail edge.) Fresh red hemorrhages, especially at the base of nail, are more important than brown linear streaks near the tips of the fingers. White-centered petechiae are most easily seen on the conjunctiva of the everted lower lid.
         c. Osler's nodes (painful, tender, reddish-brown raised areas 3–15 mm in diameter, occasionally with a whitish center, on the palms or soles).
         d. Janeway lesions (painless, circular or oval, pink to tan macules about 5 mm in diameter on the palms and soles that do not blanch with pressure).

7. What cardiac condition is suggested by brownish, muddy pigmentation of the skin and signs of hepatic failure, such as loss of axillary and pubic hair?

   ANS: Hemochromatosis with a cardiomyopathy due to intracellular iron deposits in the heart muscle, with secondary interstitial fibrosis.

8. When can amyloid disease with cardiac involvement cause skin lesions? What kind of lesions?

   ANS: Only if it is primary or if it is secondary to multiple myeloma, i.e., not if it is secondary to infection. Yellowish brown papules, nodules, or plaques may develop, often pruritic, with signs of bleeding due to scratching.

9. What is livedo reticularis? What is its significance?

   ANS: The term indicates a marbling reticulation or fishnet type of mottling of the lower trunk, buttocks, and extremities, precipitated or exaggerated by cold or by emotional upsets. It occurs in about 20% of patients with lupus erythematosus, periarteritis nodosa, or cryoglobulinemia. If it has occurred recently in a man over age 50, it suggests cholesterol embolization from an abdominal aortic aneurysm [1].

10. What are the cutaneous manifestations of intestinal **carcinoid** disease? What are the cardiac manifestations?

    ANS: The face and neck may show various blends of red and purple, often patchy and mottled. If the disease has been present for a long time, telangiectasia may be present, as may pulmonary or tricuspid stenosis and regurgitation caused by fibrosis of valve structures.

11. What diagnosis can be made by noting facial flushing following a syncopal attack?

   ANS: A cardiac arrest or a **Stokes-Adams attack**. The flush is probably a manifestation of the total-body reactive hyperemia that follows a temporary cessation of circulation.

12. What conditions that can affect the heart, besides thyrotoxicosis, can cause warmer-than-average skin?

   ANS: Severe anemia and beer drinkers' acute **beriberi**.

13. What kind of conditions are suggested by cold hands and feet?

   ANS: a. If hands and feet are moist, they suggest anxiety and may explain chest pains, palpitations, and fatigue as seen in **neurocirculatory asthenia** (DaCosta's syndrome).

   b. If only the feet are cold and the patient has a history of **intermittent claudication**, peripheral arterial obstruction with poor collateral circulation is suggested.

   c. If cold extremities are relatively recent in onset (a few weeks to a few years), a low output state is suggested.

   Note: The cold hands of the low output state can become warm when palmar erythema (liver palms) develops, secondary to cardiac cirrhosis.

14. What are the skin signs of pheochromocytoma of adrenals?

   ANS: Neurofibromatosis, cafe-au-lait spots, and axillary freckling (Crowe's sign).

CONGENITAL AND ACQUIRED FACIES

1. What are the facies of supravalvular aortic stenosis, also known as Williams syndrome?

   ANS.: A flattened occiput, broad high forehead, puffy cheeks, low ears, ocular **hypertelorism** with strabimus, underdeveloped nasal bones, an upturned nose with a long filtrum (the vertical groove between nose and mouth), a wide pouting mouth, dental abnormalities, and hypoplastic mandible. Patients commonly have atrial and/or ventricular septal defects.

2. What are the facies of Down syndrome (trisomy 21)? What are the cardiac abnormalities?

   ANS: A flattened occiput, disproportionately small head, epicanthal folds that give the impression of slanted eyes, and a mouth held open by a large protruding tongue. The most common cardiac abnormalities are various combinations of **atrial septal defects**, **ventricular septal defects**,

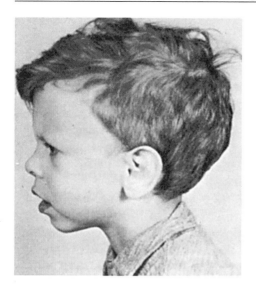 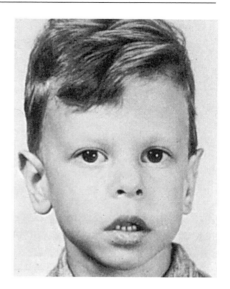

This boy with severe supravalvular aortic stenosis does not have all its facial characteristics; e.g., there is no hypertelorism or strabismus.

and atrioventricular (AV) valve regurgitation due to various degrees of **endocardial cushion defects**.

3. What is de Musset's sign?

    ANS: Head-nodding movements secondary to the ballistic force of severe aortic regurgitation (AR).

    Note: The sign was named after a patient, Alfred de Musset, a French poet whose nodding movements were described by his brother in a biography.

4. What are the facies of myxedema? What cardiac abnormalities are expected?

    ANS: Puffy lids and loss of the outer third of the eyebrows: scanty, dry, hair; coarse, dry skin; expressionless face, and an enlarged tongue.

    Note: These patients have cardiomyopathies due to increased interstitial fluid and mucoid infiltration. They also have pericardial effusions.

5. What is meant by an earlobe crease, and what is its significance?

    ANS: This is an oblique crease in the earlobe. Ninety percent of patients over age 50 with significant triple vessel coronary disease have a deep earlobe crease. A unilateral ear crease was found in one study to be associated with an intermediate degree of coronary obstruction [2]. (See p. 22.)

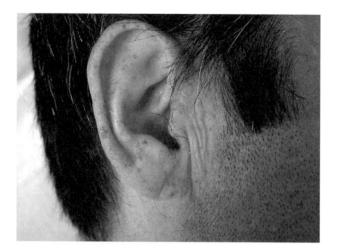

This 47-year-old man had this deep ear crease bilaterally. Although he had no significant coronary disease, his cholesterol-to-HDL ratio was 8 to 1, and he had sinus node dysfunction. He was about 50 lb overweight.

6. What is the malar flush?

　　ANS: Cyanotic cheeks with a slight telangiectasia. It was once thought to be specific for mitral stenosis, pulmonary hypertension, and high venous pressure. However, it can be seen in any patient with low cardiac output and high venous pressure. It can also be seen in those who lead an outdoor life, as well as in patients with myxedema. It is sometimes seen in patients with severe pulmonary stenosis with atrial septal defects and cushingoid moon facies, as well as in the carcinoid syndrome.

　　　　　In systemic lupus, the cheeks will also be reddened, but with a butterfly erythema that covers the cheeks and bridge of the nose. In these patients lesions are also found in exposed areas such as the scalp, external auditory canal, neck, and upper chest. The heart may be involved in lupus with pericarditis, myocarditis, Libman-Sacks verrucous endocarditis of the mitral or aortic valve, and occasional myocardial infarction due to coronary arteritis.

EYES

1. What is the cardiac cause of jaundice?

　　ANS: Jaundice may be a sign of severe heart failure, with high venous pressure causing liver damage.

2. Which kind of corneal arcus (circumferential light gray or yellowish ring around the rim of the iris) is associated with hypercholesterolemia or coronary disease?

　　ANS: A thick band that begins inferiorly and is inside the limbus, allowing a thin rim of iris pigment to be seen between the arcus and the sclera. The

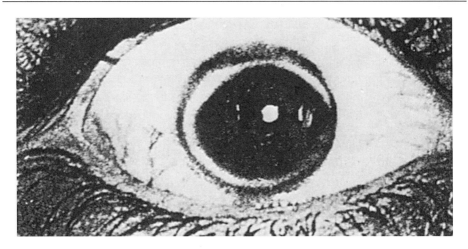

This type of arcus is a thick band of yellowish material surrounded by peripheral pigment and suggests a high serum cholesterol. It is not an arcus senilis, which has little known significance. (Courtesy Ayerst Laboratories.)

usual "arcus senilis" is not necessarily associated with hyperlipidemia or coronary disease. It begins superiorly and extends to the rim or limbus of the iris.

3. How does **infective endocarditis** affect the eyes?

   ANS: a. Conjunctival hemorrhages and petechiae (due to tendency to bleed plus minute emboli). Evert lids to see these lesions.

   b. Oval or canoe-shaped hemorrhages near optic disk with white spot in center (Roth spots).

4. With which cardiac lesions are cataracts associated?

   ANS: They may be part of the rubella syndrome in which a PDA and pulmonary artery (not valve) stenosis are the most common cardiac lesions. Other features may include deafness and mental deficiency due to microcephaly. The rate of growth may be slow.

5. Which cardiac lesion should you suspect in the presence of an Argyll Robertson pupil (reacts to accommodation but not to light)?

   ANS: Luetic aortic aneurysm or luetic AR with coronary ostial stenosis.

6. Which cardiac condition besides thyrotoxic heart disease may be associated with exophthalmos?

   ANS: Advanced congestive heart failure with high venous pressure and weight loss. The stare is probably due to lid retraction caused by the strong sympathetic tone accompanying the low cardiac output, and exaggerated by the slight proptosis.

7. What cardiac lesions should you suspect if you see a tremulous iris (iridodonesis) when gaze shifts rapidly from side to side?

   ANS: This sign suggests the Marfan syndrome, in which the iris is not properly supported by the lens because of dislocation or weakness of the suspensory ligament. The cardiac lesions associated with it are aneurysms of the aorta or pulmonary artery and myxomatous degeneration of the aorta or mitral valve, with consequent regurgitation.

8. What is the significance of xanthelasma (flat **xanthomas** or yellowish cholesterol-filled plaque on or around the eyelid)?

   ANS: It is usually associated with hypercholesterolemia.

9. What are the retinal signs of various degrees of **arteriosclerosis** [3]?

   ANS: Grade 1:   The light reflex is increased in width.

   Grade 2:   Crossing abnormalities (arteriovenous nicking and right-angled crossing of the arteries over the veins).

   Grade 3:   Copper-wire arteries (red color of artery is slightly brownish due to thick walls).

   Grade 4:   Silver-wire arteries (no red color is seen, only a whitish light reflex).

   Note: Hollenhorst plaques are flakes of cholesterol emboli seen as glinting spots, often seeming larger than the vessels in which they reside.

10. What are the retinal signs of different degrees of hypertension?

    ANS: Grade 1:   Generalized attenuation (arteriovenous ratio of less than 2 to 3).

    Grade 2:   Focal constriction or spasm.

    Grade 3:   Hemorrhages and exudates. (Exudates may either resemble cotton wool or be hard and shiny.)

    Grade 4:   Papilledema.

    Note: Pure attenuation of the arterioles is best seen in toxemia of pregnancy or in young persons with rapid onset of hypertension. Minimal narrowing is most easily seen beyond the first or second bifurcation where the arteries actually become arterioles. Corkscrew tortuosity with frequent "U turns" may be seen with coarctation and sometimes with retinal hemorrhages.

11. What three cardiac conditions are associated with a blue sclera?

    ANS: a. Osteogenesis imperfecta is associated with AR.
          b. The Marfan syndrome is associated with great-vessel aneurysms and mitral or aortic valve regurgitation.

       c. Ehlers-Danlos syndrome, with its hyperelastic, fragile skin, hyperextensible joints, and kyphoscoliosis, is associated with atrial septal defect (ASD), tetralogy of Fallot, or regurgitant valves.

12. What are angioid streaks?

     ANS: Brown linear streaks perpendicular to blood vessels. Seen in pseudoxanthoma elasticum and endocardial fibrosis and regurgitation in the heart.

EDEMA

1. How can you demonstrate edema even when it is slight?

     ANS: Press on the skin over a bony area for 10 s with at least three fingers spread slightly apart, and feel for valleys between hills after release.

2. What is the significance of slow and fast edema?

     ANS: With slow edema, the pitting remains for more than 1 min, and it is most likely due to congestion. If, however, the pitting disappears in less than 40 s (fast edema), the cause is almost certainly a low albumin level [4]. (The venous pressure presumably controls the rate of tissue fluid flow from the legs.)

3. What are the usual causes of noncardiac bilateral leg edema, besides low albumin?

     ANS: a. Premenstrual edema (hormonal).

          b. Tight undergarments.

          c. Obesity (obstructed lymphatics).

4. How can you rule out a cardiac cause for the edema?

     ANS: Check the venous pressure. Normal venous pressure is incompatible with a cardiac cause of the edema unless diuretics have been given. Face and hand edema tend to rule out a cardiac cause except in infants.

5. Where should you check for edema in a bedridden patient?

     ANS: Only presacral edema may be present if the patient has been in bed for some time.

6. How much body fluid may collect in tissue before pitting occurs?

     ANS: At least 10 lb (4.5 kg).

7. How can you tell that ascites is present?

     ANS.: If flanks are resonant, swelling is probably gas, common in severe congestive heart failure (CHF). If ascites is from CHF, the liver is enlarged and often ballotable.

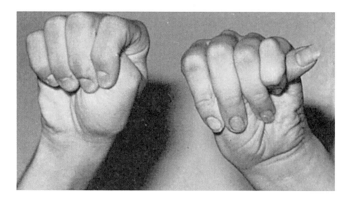

At left is a normal subject, who is unable to protrude his thumb beyond his clenched fingers, as can the patient with the Marfan syndrome at right, who can do this because of a long thumb and lax joints.

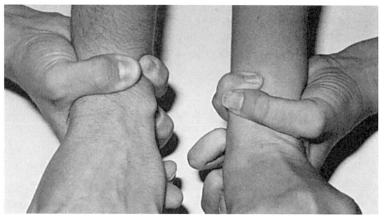

The normal patient at left cannot overlap his thumb and little finger around his wrist because, unlike the patient with the Marfan syndrome at right, his fingers are not long relative to his wrist.

EXTREMITIES

1. What hand, wrist, and extremity findings suggest the Marfan syndrome, with its possible cardiac abnormalities of aortic regurgitation and prolapsed mitral valve?

    ANS: a. Fingers: slender and long ("spider" fingers, or arachnodactyly).

    b. Thumb sign: when a fist is made over a clenched thumb, the thumb should not extend beyond the ulnar side of the hand. (False positives of this sign occur in 1% of white children and 3% of African American children.)

    c. Wrist sign: when the wrist is encircled by the thumb and the little finger (with light pressure), the little finger will overlap at least 1 cm in 80% of patients with the Marfan syndrome.

    d. The span of the outstretched arms exceeds the height by at least 5 cm.

2. What is the most common cardiac lesion associated with rheumatoid arthritis?

    ANS: Pericarditis and even occasional constrictive pericarditis.

3. What skeletal abnormalities suggest an atrial septal defect (ASD)?

    ANS: a. Any skeletal deformity of the Marfan syndrome suggests not only pulmonary artery or aortic dilatation but also an ASD.

          b. A prominent left precordium suggests not only that the right ventricle (RV) was dilated during childhood but also that it was working against a high pressure. This deformity suggests that the ejection murmur is due to an ASD with hyperkinetic pulmonary hypertension.

          c. A thumb deformity such as a fingerlike thumb (three phalanges) or an extra-short thumb, combined with an ASD, is called the Holt-Oram syndrome. An ulnar-radial deformity that prevents good forearm supination or pronation may be present with this syndrome.

4. What cardiovascular abnormality is associated with Turner's syndrome?

    ANS: Coarctation.

5. What are the hand signs of Down's syndrome, besides the simian crease?

    ANS.: The fourth and fifth fingers are abnormally separated and the fifth finger is short and curved inward.

CHEST AND RESPIRATION

1. Which cardiac abnormalities are suggested by a **pectus excavatum**?

    ANS: a. This may occur in the Marfan syndrome, with aortic or pulmonary artery aneurysms, or myxomatous degeneration of the mitral or aortic valve with regurgitation. An ASD should also be suspected. (Pectus carinatum, or pigeon breast, may also occur with the Marfan syndrome.)

          b. It may be part of the straight-back syndrome (see Chapter 13).

2. What should **Cheyne-Stokes respiration** suggest in a cardiac patient?

    ANS.: A very low output at rest. The anoxic respiratory center becomes insensitive to normal tensions of CO_2. The apnea causes hypercapnea, which stimulates the respiratory center, resulting in hyperpnea, which washes out the CO_2 and apnea recurs.

3. What is the significance of a short breath-holding time?

    ANS: It signifies either

          a. Chronic hyperventilation, or

          b. Poor psychophysical control of the breathing apparatus. The normal subject (with legs dangling) can hold his or her breath for 30 s

with a little encouragement. Inability to hold it for at least 20 s is
abnormal and can explain dyspnea on exertion. Heart failure or
chronic obstructive pulmonary disease (COPD) does not shorten
breath-holding time unless there is dyspnea at rest.

4. What is a shield chest, and what does it suggest?

ANS: It is a broad chest with a greater angle than usual between the manubrium and the body of the sternum, as well as widely separated nipples.
In a female with neck webbing, wide carrying angle, and short stature
(under 5 ft in height) it suggests **Turner's syndrome** and concomitant
coarctation. In a male it is called Noonan's or Ullrich's syndrome and is
commonly associated with pulmonary stenosis.

5. What is Ewart's sign of a large pericardial effusion?

ANS.: Compression of the lung results in a patch of marked dullness between
the angle of the left scapula and the spine, associated with tubular (bronchial) breathing and egophany in the same area.

6. How can crackles (formerly called rales) help diagnose lung abnormalities?

ANS.: Paninspiratory: pneumonia or CHF. Early: severe COPD, asthma or
chronic bronchitis. Late: interstitial edema, pulmonary fibrosis, or
resolving CHF. Early to mid: bronchiectasis.

Note: Most crackles are not due to CHF but due to sputum in the air passages
which often disappear with several coughs. In early CHF crackles may
be absent.

REFERENCES

1. Kazmier, F. J., et al. Livedo reticularis and digital infarcts: A syndrome due to cholesterol emboli arising from atheromatous abdominal aortic aneurysms. *Cardio. Comp.*
1:56, 1966.
2. Lichstein, E., et al. Diagonal ear-lobe crease and coronary artery sclerosis. *Ann.
Intern. Med.* 85:337, 1976.
3. Scheie, H. G. Evaluation of ophthalmoscopic changes of hypertension and arteriolar
sclerosis. *Arch. Ophthalmol.* 49:117,1953.
4. Henry, J. A., and Altmann, P. Assessment of hypoproteinaemic oedema: A simple
physical sign. *Br. Med. J.* 1:890,1978.

3 Arterial Pulses and Pressures

METHOD OF ARM PALPATION

1. Why is palpating both brachial and radial arteries simultaneously an efficient method of palpating the arm pulses, besides speeding up the palpation of the pulses?

   ANS: It allows you to estimate the systolic blood pressure without a stethoscope or blood pressure cuff. This procedure is described later in this chapter.

   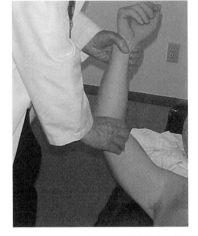

   Since the brachial artery is a medial vessel, it should be approached medially. The radial artery is a lateral vessel and therefore should be approached laterally.

2. Where are brachial arteries best sought (a) in the young patient and (b) in the older patient?

   ANS: a. In the young patient the brachial artery may be hidden just under the biceps.
   b. In the older patient brachial tortuosity tends to displace the artery medially away from the biceps.

3. What questions must you answer as you palpate a peripheral pulse?

   ANS: a. Is the rate of rise slow, normal, or fast?
   b. Is there a shoulder on the upstroke or a midsystolic dip, shoulder, or thrill?
   c. Is the pulse volume or pressure small, normal, or large?
   d. Is the vessel hard, i.e., does it roll too easily under the fingers?

e. What is the blood pressure? (For the method of estimating blood pressure by palpation, see p. 39.)

RATES OF RISE AND PULSE VOLUME

1. How can you recognize a normal rate of rise and volume of a carotid or brachial pulse?

    ANS: It feels like a gentle tap against the finger tips.

    Note: In subjects over age 45, the tap is often followed by a slower rise. The initial tap is caused by a rapid rise to a peak known as the percussion wave. The slower rise following it is called a tidal wave. The tidal wave results from waves reflected from areas where arteries divide. The fusion of reflected and percussion waves forms the tidal waves.

2. What is the shoulder produced by the change in slope of the carotid upstroke seen in elderly subjects called?

    ANS: The anacrotic shoulder

    Note: Since pulse rises become more rapid as you palpate more peripherally, the shoulder may disappear by the time the pulse reaches the brachials or even high in the neck in comparison with low in the neck.

The normal percussion wave (first peak) is felt as a sharp tap. In the older age groups an anacrotic shoulder occurs, resulting in a late tidal wave that is felt as further outward motion after the initial tap. More peripherally, the shoulder to a higher tidal wave disappears. A shoulder on the upstroke of a percussion wave feels like a "tap and push" effect.

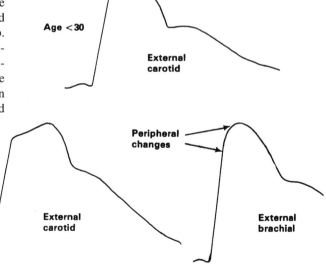

Slow Rate of Rise

1. What is the sensation to the fingers when there is a slow rate of rise? Why?

    ANS: The first indication that the rise is slow is the absence of a tap. Then you may notice that the sensation is one of a caressing lift, a gentle push, or a nudge. If you feel a tap followed by a push, then you may be feeling an anacrotic shoulder followed by a late slow-rising tidal wave.

The normal rise is a tap; the slow rise is a caress.

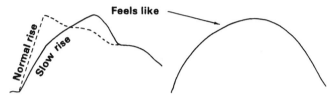

2. What is the significance of a slow rate of rise in the carotid pulse?

    ANS: It tells you that there is probably **aortic stenosis** (AS) due to fixed obstruction to aortic flow.

3. On which side of the neck is the carotid murmur of AS more likely to be palpated?

    ANS: A thrill may be palpated more often over the left carotid than on the right.

    Note: A lag between the onset of the apical impulse and the carotid impulse predicts a valve area of less than 1 cm^2 (100% specific).

If an almost normal tap is followed by a sustained thrill, this is the plateau pulse of AS. In the above figure L_2 = lead 2, and 2 RIS means that the microphone was in the second right interspace.

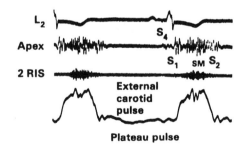

Plateau pulse

Severity of Aortic Stenosis by Rates of Rise

1. How does the peripheral increase of rate of rise affect an anacrotic shoulder or slow rise of mild AS?

    ANS: The anacrotic shoulder and a slow rise in the carotid may become a normal rate of rise in the brachials. However, if myocardial function is decreased, the slow rise of even mild AS may be transmitted to the brachials.

Boldface type indicates that the term is explained in the glossary.

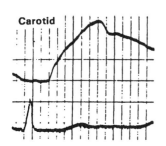 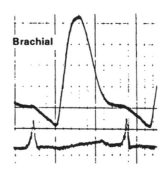

Carotid and brachial pulse contours in a patient with mild AS. By the time the pulse wave reached the brachials, it had become normal.

2. How does the rigid aorta of severe **arteriosclerosis** in the elderly affect the carotid rate of rise in the presence of AS?

    ANS: There may be a normal rate of rise in the carotids. This phenomenon is presumably due to the inability of a noncompliant aorta to expand slowly [1].

3. Why does supravalvular AS have both rate of rise and blood pressure greater on the right carotid and subclavian than on the left?

    ANS: Because there is streaming of the jet straight up along the ascending aorta toward the innominate, right carotid, and right subclavian arteries.

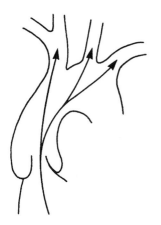 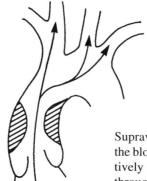

Supravalvular obstruction caused the blood in the aorta to take a relatively sharp turn before it can exit through the left carotid and subclavian arteries.

Rapid Rates of Rise (Brisk Pulse) with Normal Pulse Pressures

1. When will a large volume ejected from the left ventricle (LV) have a normal pulse pressure?

    ANS: If there are two outlet orifices for ejection, as in mitral regurgitation (MR) or **ventricular septal defect** (VSD).

2. Why is there an increase in volume in the LV in MR and VSD?

   ANS: In MR and VSD the LV receives two sources of blood in diastole. In MR, the LV receives the normal amount from the left atrium plus the blood it regurgitated in the previous systole. In VSD, the LV receives, in addition to the normal left atrial blood, the blood it shunted into the RV and pulmonary circuit in the previous systole.

This depicts the extra diastolic flow through the mitral valve that takes place when MR occurs during the previous ventricular systole. In MR, the normal pulmonary venous return to the LV is added to the returning regurgitant flow to increase the volume in the LV beyond normal. Thus, in MR, the left artrium is volume-overloaded during ventricular systole and the LV is volume-overloaded during ventricular diastole.

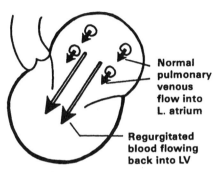

Normal pulmonary venous flow into L. atrium

Regurgitated blood flowing back into LV

Note that the arrows representing ejection into the aorta are equal, i.e., the forward stroke volume in MR is not reduced unless the MR is very severe or there is cardiac damage.

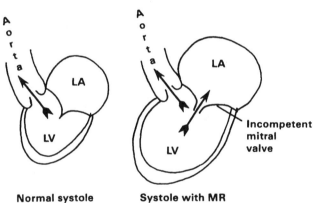

Incompetent mitral valve

Normal systole   **Systole with MR**

3. Why is the pulse rise brisk in MR and VSD volume overloads?

   ANS: The increased volume produces a **Starling effect** on the LV.

4. Why is there a brisk rate of rise with hypertrophic obstructive cardiomyopathy (HOCM)?

   ANS: In HOCM there is no obstruction until the outflow tract contracts and approximates the thickened septum to a mitral leaflet. Because of a catecholamine effect on the hypertrophied muscle, the LV ejects as much as 80% of its blood before the obstruction occurs. The rate of rise in HOCM is among the fastest in cardiology.

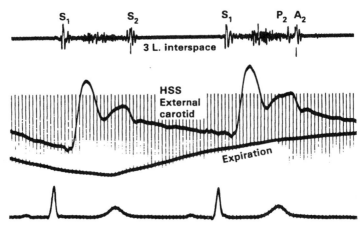

This is a phonocardiogram and pulse tracing from a 34-year-old woman with HOCM. The outflow gradient was 70 mmHg. Some mitral regurgitation was present. There was a large LV on X-ray. Note the rapid rate of rise to a high percussion wave and the midsystolic dip that produce the "pointed-finger" carotid pulse contour.

5. What is the Brockenbrough effect?

    ANS: In normal subjects the postextrasystolic pulse after a long pause is larger than normal. In HOCM it appears to stay the same because of the increase in obstruction due to the Starling effect, the **postextrasystolic potentiation** effect and the decrease in afterload, all causing an increase in contractility.

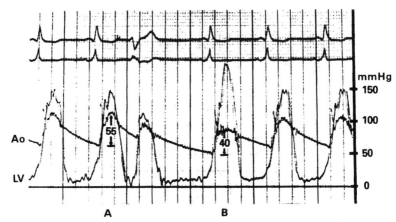

The Brockenbrough effect is seen in the postextrasystolic beat B because the pulse pressure decreased to 40 mmHg from 55 mmHg during sinus rhythm at A.

Rapid Rates of Rise with Increased Pulse Pressure

1. What name is given to describe a rapidly rising pulse with an increased pulse volume or pulse pressure?

   ANS: Bounding

2. What are the most common cardiac causes of a bounding pulse?

   ANS: Aortic regurgitation (AR), **persistent ductus arteriosus**, and coarctation.

3. What are the most common noncardiac causes of a rapid rise with increased pulse pressure?

   ANS: Thyrotoxicosis, pregnancy, and severe anemia.

4. Why is the pulse of AR bounding?

   ANS: a. There is a high systolic pressure because a large volume is ejected. The large volume is from two sources: the diastolic AR flow plus the mitral diastolic flow. The Starling effect caused by stretching the LV creates the rapid rise.

   b. There is a low diastolic pressure.

5. What causes the decreased diastolic pressure in AR?

   ANS: The lower diastolic pressure in AR is only partly due to backflow into the LV during systole. It is mostly due to the reflex decrease in peripheral resistance caused by the large stroke volume stretching the carotid and aortic sinuses. Although gross AR will generally have a diastolic pressure of about 50 mmHg or less, if the patient goes into heart failure the resultant reflex increase in peripheral resistance caused by low output may raise the diastolic pressure to normal values.

This illustration represents ventricular diastole in a patient with AR. The reason for the large volume in diastole in AR is obvious, since the LV fills from two sources. As long as the LV is healthy, it will eject the usual 60–75% of its increased end-diastolic volume, i.e., its ejection fraction will remain normal. Thus, the aorta will receive a large stroke volume with each systole.

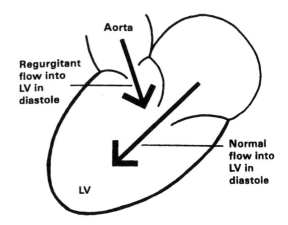

6. How can you exaggerate the rapid rate of rise and increased pulse pressure in AR?

   ANS: Elevate the patient's arm as you feel the radial artery with the distal palmar surface of your hand. You will find that a larger pulse volume occurs only if the patient has significant AR.

   Note: If the diastolic pressure as measured by the arm elevated vertically is over 15 mm lower than that measured by the arm in the conventional position, aortic regurgitation is probably present.

7. What is Corrigan's pulse?

   ANS: It is the bounding carotid seen by eye.

   Note: a. The large volume and rapidly rising pulse of AR detected by palpation is often called a water-hammer pulse. A water hammer, a Victorian toy, consists of a vacuum tube partly filled with water. When the tube is inverted, the water drops like a rock due to unopposed gravity and strikes the bottom of the tube with a loud noise.

   b. The loud sounds heard when the stethoscope is placed over the rapidly rising large pulsations of the femoral artery are called Traube's sign, or pistol-shot sounds.

8. What is Duroziez' double murmur?

   ANS: Duroziez' double murmur consists of two murmurs: the first is the systolic murmur heard by gradually compressing the femoral artery with a finger proximal to the stethoscope chest piece; the second is a diastolic murmur produced by gradually compressing the artery distal to the stethoscope. This latter murmur is due to backflow as the blood in all the large arteries flows backward toward the aortic valve in diastole.

   Note: Traub's sign and Duroziez' double murmurs are more of historical than practical interest because no more information is gained from them than by palpating the pulses or taking a blood pressure.

Summary of Quick Diagnoses Possible from the Carotid Pulse

1. Feel for a gentle tap. This means you are feeling a carotid with a normal amplitude and rate of rise. (Feel your own carotid with light to moderate finger pressure to learn what a normal pulse volume with a normal rate of rise feels like.)

2. If you feel no tap but only a "push" you should assume that aortic stenosis is probably present.

3. If you feel a sharp tap (brisk pulse) due to a rapid rate of rise, consider MR, VSD, or HCM if the pulse volume or pressure is normal. If the pulse amplitude is increased, consider AR, PDA, or coarctation.

PULSUS BISFERIENS

1. What is meant by a bisferiens pulse?

    ANS: *Bis* means "twice" and *feriens* means "beating." Therefore, a bisferiens pulse is a twice-beating pulse. Actually it is a double-peaked arterial pulse so that there is a midsystolic dip in systole.

2. What is the physiological significance of a bisferiens pulse?

    ANS: It is always associated with the ejection of a rapid jet of blood through the aortic valve. At the peak of flow, a Bernoulli effect (suction effect of rapid flow over a surface) on the walls of the ascending aorta causes a sudden decrease in lateral pressure on the inner aspect of the wall.

3. What causes the most marked bisferiens pulse?

    ANS: A combination of moderate AS and severe AR [2].

The fall in lateral wall pressure during peak velocity requires a high velocity of ejection. This implies the presence of a relatively healthy myocardium.

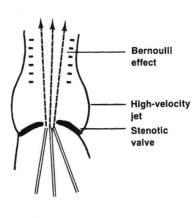

AS + AR

4. When can AS cause a bisferiens pulse in the absence of AR?

    ANS: Severe HOCM can have a bisferiens pulse. (See p. 38)

    Note: a. A carotid shudder describes a short vibration effect when AS and AR produces a slight bisferiens effect, and suggests that there is no significant myocardial depression. Pure severe AR can produce either a carotid thrill or bisferiens pulse.

    b. A double-peaked systolic wave is sometimes more easily felt in the brachial or radial artery than in the carotid.

    c. A bisferiens pulse is more likely in younger patients, perhaps because the arterial tree is more distensible.

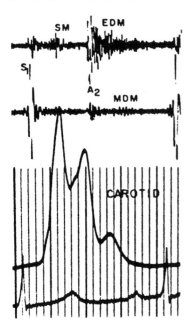

Bisferiens pulse in a patient with severe AR. (EDM = early diastolic murmur of AR at left sternal border; MDM = mid-diastolic murmur at apex [Austin Flint murmur]).

The Palpable Dicrotic Wave

1. What is a dicrotic wave?

    ANS: A dicrotic wave is a small wave that follows the dicrotic notch in an external carotid pressure tracing. On auscultation, S_2 separates the two components of the dicrotic pulse.

    Note: The dicrotic notch is the notch on a carotid pulse tracing at the time of aortic valve closure. The same notch in an aortic pressure tracing is called the incisura.

PALPATION OF THE LEG PULSES

1. What are some of the points to help you feel difficult popliteals with the patient supine?

    ANS: a. Popliteals are never directly palpable. You should only attempt to feel their transmitted pulsations.

    b. Maintain similar sensations of skin to skin on all parts of the palms of both hands by having the palms in complete contact with the patient's skin, i.e., there should be no air separating any of your hand from the patient's skin.

    c. Squeeze with the entire hand, i.e., with the thumbs as well as with the fingers.

2. How can you best feel a faint posterior tibial or dorsalis pedis pulse?

    ANS: Try various degrees of dorsiflexion of the foot in order to separate the extensor retinaculum of the ankle from the arteries.

3. Where is the usual site to find a palpable dorsalis pedis?

    ANS: Between the great and index toes.

    Note: a. The dorsalis pedis may be absent in as many as 10% of normal adults.

    b. The main purpose of palpating the foot pulses routinely is to document the foot pulses as a basis for future follow-up of peripheral vascular problems.

    c. If the skin of the foot is colder than expected and the leg pulses smaller than expected, elevate each leg passively. This intensifies the pallor in the ischemic limb, with little effect on the limb with normal arterial circulation.

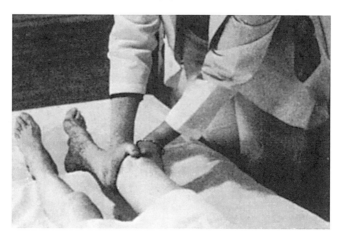

It will not be necessary to place the patient in the prone position if you remember that the key to popliteal palpation is to feel for an area of transmitted pulsation.

ESTIMATING SYSTOLIC BLOOD PRESSURE BY PALPATION ALONE

1. If it takes only gentle pressure on a brachial artery to obliterate the ipsilateral radial that you are palpating simultaneously, what is the systolic pressure?

    ANS: Almost certainly normal, i.e., about 120 ± 20 mmHg. This assumes that the pulse volume in the radials is not so small that they already are almost impalpable.

2. What is the systolic pressure if it takes (a) moderate or (b) marked pressure on the brachials to obliterate the radials?

    ANS: a. The blood pressure is probably between 130 and 160 mmHg.

                b. The blood pressure may be over 160 mmHg.

   Note: a. A reliable estimation can only be made when gentle pressure eliminates the radials, because there are too many factors to consider if it takes more than slight pressure to obliterate the radials.

                b. You can eliminate the confusing effect of pushing a brachial into a groove by carrying out the procedure on the opposite arm.

ACCURATE BLOOD PRESSURE MEASUREMENT

1. How do the heart and blood vessels control arterial systolic and diastolic pressure levels?

    ANS: Systolic blood pressure (the highest pressure reached by the arteries) is controlled by the stroke volume of the heart and the stiffness of the arterial vessels that receive the stroke volume. Diastolic blood pressure (lowest pressure found in the aorta and its branches after maximal runoff into the periphery) is controlled primarily by peripheral resistance.

2. What is normal systolic and diastolic blood pressure?

    ANS: In an adult the upper limit of normal blood pressure should probably be considered to be 140/90 mmHg.

   Note: A rough rule of thumb for systolic pressure in infants and children is:

$$90 + \frac{(\text{age in years} \times 5)}{3}$$

3. What arterial abnormality can cause a rise in systolic blood pressure and leave diastolic blood pressure normal?

    ANS: A stiff aorta, secondary to atherosclerosis in elderly patients.

   Note: It used to be taught that an elevated diastolic pressure is more associated with a poor cardiovascular prognosis than an elevated systolic pressure. It is now known that an elevated systolic pressure has the same or a worse prognosis than an increase in diastolic pressure, because of the harmful effects of an increase in pulse pressure.

4. In what percentage of patients is there a difference of 10 mmHg or more in *systolic* blood pressure between the arms if the pressure in both arms is taken separately?

    ANS: If hypertensives are included, 25% of patients will have at least a 10-mmHg difference in systolic blood pressure [3]. If only normotensive patients are studied, only about 1% will have a 10-mmHg difference.

5. If a patient has a history of presyncope or syncope on standing (orthostatic hypotension), how long should the patient stand before checking for a fall in blood pressure?

    ANS: If the blood pressure does not fall immediately, you should recheck after 3–5 min of standing.

    Note: A drop of more than 15 mmHg in systolic pressure or any fall in diastolic pressure suggests hypovolemia or autonomic dysfunction.

KOROTKOFF SOUNDS

1. What is meant by Korotkoff sounds?

    ANS: these are sounds produced by the pulsations of an artery under a partially constricting blood pressure cuff (described by the Russian physician N. S. Korotkoff in 1905).

2. What are the conventional five phases of Korotkoff sounds, and which ones are the only important ones to remember?

    ANS: The five phases are: phase 1, onset of tapping sounds; phase 2, at a pressure of about 10–15 mmHg lower than phase 1, a murmur may be heard after the tap; phase 3, reappearance of only the tapping sound; phase 4, muffling; phase 5, disappearance of sounds. Phases 4 and 5, i.e., muffling and disappearance, are the only phases that are sometimes referred to in the literature by numbers.

3. By how much may blood pressure be wrong if the Korotkoff sounds are soft?

    ANS: By as much as 60 mmHg.

4. How can you increase the loudness of Korotkoff sounds?

    ANS: a. Increase brachial flow by having the patient open and clench the fist about 10 times. If popliteal or foot pressures are being taken, flexion and extension of the ankle serves the same purpose. This degree of mild exercise does not alter the actual blood pressure.

    b. Inflate the cuff quickly.

    c. Elevate the arm before inflating the cuff.

    Note: Steps a and b above should be done routinely, and step c should be done only if the Korotkoff sounds are still soft.

5. Why will rapid cuff inflation increase loudness of Korotkoff sounds?

    ANS: Slow inflation prolongs the low pressure phases of inflation, which acts as a venous tourniquet and traps venous blood in the forearm. The increased blood volume in the forearm will decrease the flow gradient of the arterial blood passing under the cuff during deflation.

6. How can you get an accurate blood pressure without a stethoscope?

   ANS: Palpate the brachial artery with a thumb at the cuff edge. The systolic pressure occurs when the pulse returns; the diastolic pressure occurs when an increasingly dynamic pulse suddenly feels normal.

CHEST PIECE PLACEMENT AND CHOICE

1. Where are Korotkoff sounds loudest? (a) In the center of the cuff, (b) at the edge of the cuff, or (c) a few centimeters distal to the cuff edge?

   ANS: In the center of the cuff.

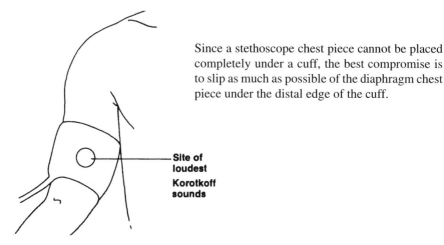

Since a stethoscope chest piece cannot be placed completely under a cuff, the best compromise is to slip as much as possible of the diaphragm chest piece under the distal edge of the cuff.

Site of loudest Korotkoff sounds

2. Are Korotkoff sounds dominantly low or high frequency?

   ANS: Low.

3. If Korotkoff sounds are dominantly low frequency, why is it better to use the diaphragm chest piece, which is designed for high frequency?

   ANS: a. A bell chest piece cannot get as close to the center of the cuff as can a diaphragm, because a piece of the diaphragm can be inserted under the cuff.

        b. A good air seal is difficult to obtain with a bell on a rounded arm surface unless firm pressure is applied. Heavy pressure with the stethoscope may result in a falsely low diastolic pressure.

4. What is the best position for the patient's arm to locate the brachial artery quickly?

   ANS: The patient's palm should face upward. In this position the brachial artery is more easily located than with the palm in any other position.

5. When is a bell chest piece preferable in taking a blood pressure?

    ANS: a. When the high frequencies in Korotkoff sounds disappear, as when a patient is in shock.

    b. When the blood pressure is recorded in the thigh with the chest piece in the popliteal space where the Korotkoff sounds are soft partly because rapid inflation of a thigh cuff is difficult.

EQUIPMENT SOURCES OF ERROR

1. It used to be taught that a mercury manometer always be used in preference to an aneroid (rotating-needle) type. Is this still true?

    ANS: About 15% of hospital aneroid manometers are inaccurate by about 10 mmHg when tested against a mercury manometer. The error can be in the low, middle, or upper pressure range. However, there is now a shift back to using aneroid manometers (with frequent testing against mercury manometers) because of the occasional danger of mercury poisoning should the manometer break.

2. What is the effect of a too-narrow cuff on the blood pressure reading?

    ANS: A too-narrow cuff may require excessive inflation pressure to occlude the brachial artery. As a result, the pressure reading may be as much as 50 mmHg too high.

3. What is considered to be an adequate cuff width relative to the arm diameter or circumference for obtaining an accurate blood pressure?

    ANS: The cuff width (not length) should be at least 40% of the arm's circumference.

    Note: a. The center of the rubber bladder must be placed over the brachial artery.

    b. The error will be less if the cuff is slightly larger than recommended than if the cuff is slightly smaller.

4. How can you overcome the small-cuff problem if a large cuff is not available for a fat arm?

    ANS: Place the cuff on the forearm and either auscultate or use a Doppler probe over the radial artery.

5. What error is likely with a loosely applied cuff?

    ANS: The pressure may be falsely high.

SYSTOLIC PRESSURE MEASUREMENT

1. Why is it usually taught that you should first inflate the cuff until you feel the radial pulse disappear?

   ANS: It is said that this will:

      a. Prevent inflating the cuff higher than necessary.
      b. Avoid being fooled by the auscultatory gap.

2. What is meant by the auscultatory gap?

   ANS: It is the silence caused by the disappearance of Korotkoff sounds after the first appearance of the true systolic pressure, and the reappearance of pressure some 10–20 mmHg lower.

3. Why is it unnecessary to feel the radial pulse disappear first before applying the stethoscope?

   ANS: a. An auscultatory gap requires venous distention of the forearm and concomitant low flow. If you routinely have the patient clench his or her fist 10 times and inflate the cuff rapidly, you will prevent the auscultatory gap [4], and the extra time required to feel the radial pulse for this purpose will be eliminated.
      b. It is just as easy to inflate the cuff until the Korotkoff sounds disappear as it is to inflate the cuff until the radial pulse disappears.

Avoiding Technical Errors in Finding Systolic Pressure

1. How high should you inflate the cuff?

   ANS: It is not necessary to inflate the cuff more than 10 mmHg above systolic pressure. Unnecessarily higher inflation may cause discomfort that may elevate blood pressure falsely, and it also makes it take longer to deflate to systolic pressure. In adults, you may immediately raise the cuff pressure to 140 mmHg and listen for Korotkoff sounds. If Korotkoff sounds are present, then inflate another 10 mmHg and keep doing this until the Korotkoff sounds disappear. In children it is probably better to inflate immediately to only 120 mmHg. Thus, instead of taking time to feel for disappearance of the radial pulse to note the degree of cuff inflation, with the Korotkoff sound method you will never inflate more than about 10 mm Hg above systolic pressure.

2. How slowly should you deflate the cuff?

   ANS: Not more than 5 mmHg per second or per beat, especially when beginning to deflate. This will prevent deflation through the first Korotkoff sounds or through a pulsus alternans (5- to 10-mmHg difference in blood pressure in alternate beats; see below under Pulsus Alternans). Slow deflation also prevents development of a negative pressure above the mercury column.

3. Where should the brachial artery be in relation to heart level when taking blood pressure?

    ANS: The brachial artery should be at near heart level; otherwise gravity will add its pressure to the brachial artery pressure.

4. What errors occur if the rubber part of the cuff balloons beyond its covering or if the cuff is so loose that central ballooning occurs?

    ANS: Both conditions will require excessive cuff pressure to compress the artery, and the reading will be falsely high.

5. When are Doppler methods a preferable method of recording blood pressure, even though only a systolic pressure can be obtained?

    ANS: a. In infants.
    b. In legs, especially when there is arterial occlusive disease, coarctation, or a low output state.
    c. In shock states.
    d. During cardiopulmonary resuscitation (CPR) to test for effectiveness of blood flow.

    Note: The systolic blood pressure obtained by the Doppler method can be accepted as nearly the same as that obtained by a stethoscope.

6. How does taking the blood pressure in an unsupported arm over 30 s affect the blood pressure?

    ANS: The diastolic pressure may be 5 mmHg higher.

DIASTOLIC BLOOD PRESSURE RECORDING _____

1. Which is closer to intra-arterial diastolic pressure, muffling (phase 4) or disappearance (phase 5)?

    ANS: Disappearance [5].

    Note: It is also easier to get agreement between two examiners on the disappearance point than on the muffling point.

2. When must muffling be used?

    ANS: If the disappearance point is 10 mmHg or more below muffling, as in hyperkinetic states with a falsely low disappearing point. If the difference is over 10 mmHg, it is a good idea to record both muffling and disappearance, e.g., 140/70–40.

ACCURACY OF BLOOD PRESSURE RECORDING

1. Why should we round off blood pressure readings to the nearest 5 or zero digit rather than to the nearest 2?

   ANS: It is more scientific because blood pressure readings in the same patient fluctuate too much between different physicians and under different circumstances to make the last figure significant to the nearest 2. Also, it is easier to remember a number that ends with a 5 or 0. See p. 48, question 5.

   Note: a.   Most examiners record blood pressures to the nearest 2 because (1) manometers are graduated in increments of 2; (2) there is a sense of increased accuracy; (3) a definition of hypertension for treatment or insurance purposes is often based on 140/90 mmHg as being the limit of upper normal, so that 140/92 mmHg would require treatment or a change in insurance rating.

   b.   In hypertensives with ambulatory monitoring, readings vary as much as 30 mmHg during a 12-h day.

2. What are some factors that can change blood pressure beyond 2 mmHg if the blood pressure is taken by the same physician at two different times?

   ANS: a.   If the blood pressure is read during inspiration on one day and expiration on another, the readings on expiration will be slightly higher.

   b.   If blood pressures are read with the antecubital fossa at the level of the fourth parasternal interspace on one day and the xiphoid on another, the blood pressure will be about 5 mmHg higher in the xiphoid area level.

   c.   If the room is cold on one occasion and warm on another, or if the noise level is higher one time than another, the blood pressure will be slightly higher under the cooler or noisier conditions.

   d.   If the patient is under stress on one day and not on another, the readings may differ.

   e.   Because of the patient's circadian rhythm, the patient's blood pressure will be different at different times of the day. Although most patients have a lower blood pressure in the morning than in the late afternoon, by as much as 20 mmHg, individual differences exist. Untreated hypertensive patients have their highest pressures between 9:00 and 11:00 a.m.

3. What are some of the factors that can change blood pressure beyond 2 mmHg in the same patient because two different examiners have taken the blood pressure?

   ANS: a.   If one physician uses muffling and the other uses disappearance for the diastolic pressure, the readings will be different by as much as 10 mmHg.

    b. If one physician presses the chest piece harder than the other, the diastolic reading may be lower, especially if the brachial artery is soft, as in young subjects.

    c. If one physician takes the reading with the patient's arm unsupported and the other has the patient rest the arm on a table, the reading may be 5 mmHg higher in the former than in the latter.

    d. If one physician uses an aneroid manometer and the other uses a mercury manometer, the reading may be higher or lower by at least 5 mmHg.

    e. If one physician applies the cuff more loosely than the other, there may be a difference of as much as 10 mmHg.

    f. If one physician routinely inflates the cuff to almost 200 mmHg and the other to only about 20 mmHg above systolic pressure, the discomfort caused by the first physician will cause a higher systolic pressure.

    g. If one physician uses a relatively small cuff on a fat arm, and the other uses a large cuff, there may be as much as a 50-mmHg difference in pressure.

    h. If one physician's appearance and manner are threatening and the other has a more pleasant and benign personality, the patient's blood pressure may be higher by at least 5 mmHg when taken by the former.

    i. If one patient's physician takes the blood pressure with the patient sitting in a comfortable chair and the other with the patient sitting on an examining table with the legs dangling, the former will obtain a lower reading [6].

4. What are some factors that can change blood pressure beyond 2 mmHg when soft Korotkoff sounds are present?

    ANS: a. The hearing acuity of one physician may be keener than that of another.

    b. The physician who has the patient open and close his or her fist a few times to increase blood flow may hear soft Korotkoff sounds at a higher pressure than the physician who does not do this.

    c. The physician who inflates the cuff more rapidly, thus increasing blood flow to the forearm, may hear the first Korotkoff sounds at a higher reading.

    d. The physician who places the chest piece partly under the cuff will hear the faint first Korotkoff sounds sooner than one who places it 1 or 2 cm below the cuff.

    e. If there is an auscultatory gap due to low flow, the physician who knows how to increase arm flow may hear the first Korotkoff sounds at a considerably higher level than the physician who measures the blood pressure in a routine fashion.

5. What are some of the advantages of being scientific and recording the blood pressure to the nearest 5 or zero?

    ANS: a. It is easier to remember and record three rather than six numbers between each 10 mmHg (e.g., 120,125, and 130 rather than 120, 122, 124, 126,128, and 130).

           b. Estimation to the nearest 5 mmHg is also faster because the slight fluctuations of blood pressure that occur from moment to moment make it difficult and time-consuming to try to determine the pressures to the nearest 2 mmHg.

SUMMARY OF HOW TO TAKE ARM BLOOD PRESSURES BY LISTENING FOR KOROTKOFF SOUNDS _____

1. Ask the patient to extend his or her arm with the palm upward to clarify the position of the brachial artery.

2. Be sure that the center of the cuff bladder is over the brachial artery, and if you must use an aneroid manometer, make sure that the indicator needle is in the zero area on the dial before inflating the cuff.

3. Place the diaphragm of your stethoscope partly under the cuff over the brachial artery and press lightly.

4. Ask the patient to open and close the fist about 10 times.

5. Raise the cuff pressure as quickly as possible to 140 mmHg for an adult and 120 mmHg for a child with the arm at heart level, and listen for Korotkoff sounds. If they are present, pump the cuff up another 20 mmHg. Repeat the listening and pumping until no Korotkoff sounds are heard.

6. If the Korotkoff sounds are still very soft, raise the arm before inflating the cuff.

7. Deflate the cuff at a rate of about 5 mmHg per heartbeat or per second until the first Korotkoff sounds of the systolic blood pressure are heard. Record it to the nearest 5 or zero digit.

8. Listen for pulsus alternans. This requires slow cuff deflation when the first Korotkoff sound is detected.

9. Deflate the cuff further until muffling is heard. Then deflate further until the Korotkoff sounds disappear. If the difference between the muffling point and the disappearance point is less than 10 mmHg, report the disappearance point as the diastolic pressure. If, however, the difference is greater than 10 mmHg, report both numbers (to the nearest 5 or zero digit).

10. If the arm is so fat that the cuff width or bladder length is less than 40% of arm circumference, use a thigh cuff. If no thigh cuff is available, use an arm cuff over the radial artery.

PSEUDOHYPERTENSION

1. What is meant by pseudohypertension?

    ANS: Pseudohypertension refers to a misleadingly high systolic, diastolic, or mean blood pressure measured with a cuff compared with the pressure measured directly by intra-arterial needle.

2. How high a blood pressure may be recorded with "pipestem" brachial arteries secondary to medial (Monckeberg's) sclerosis with a normal intra-arterial measurement?

    ANS: More than 300 mmHg by cuff measurement, despite a reading of about 130 mmHg by intra-arterial measurement. (The diastolic pressure may also be higher by cuff measurement.)

3. When should you suspect pseudohypertension?

    ANS: The suspicion of pseudohypertension is based on the following findings. The patient is elderly and has:

    a. A blood pressure that is elevated disproportionately to the clinical findings, i.e., no evidence of LV hypertrophy on the ECG, no cardiomegaly on X-ray or physical examination, no renal failure, and no hypertensive retinopathy.
    b. A palpable radial artery after the radial pulse has been eliminated by inflation of the cuff above the systolic pressure. This is a variation of Osler's maneuver, in which he compressed the radial artery with the index finger and felt for a palpable artery distal to the site of compression.

    Note: A positive Osler test is reliable only in patients with severe hypertension.

PULSUS ALTERNANS

1. What is pulsus alternans?

    ANS: Pulsus alternans refers to an alternating fluctuation of pulse pressure, i.e., with every other beat the blood pressure is lower, presumably because of an alternation in either the number or strength of cardiac fibers contributing to each systole.

2. What is the usual etiology of pulsus alternans?

   ANS: Pulsus alternans is associated with myocardial damage. The damage is usually severe enough to cause gross heart failure. However, it may be present without heart failure when it is secondary to cardiac hypertrophy and increased afterload, as in hypertension or aortic stenosis, but with the addition of some minor myocardial damage, such as the scar of an old infarction.

3. How much alternation in blood pressure must be present between beats before alternans can be detected by palpation?

   ANS: Over 10 mmHg. However, a difference of this magnitude is unusual. Therefore, a blood pressure cuff must be used to detect a pulsus alternans by noting a sudden doubling of the Korotkoff sounds a few millimeters of mercury below the first detectable taps. Pulses alternans is easier to feel by palpation of the radial or femoral arteries than by the carotid. A very light finger pressure is necessary.

   Note: a. Palpation of the radial pulse with two fingers may be used. By varying the pressure on the proximal finger, the weaker beats can be eliminated while the stronger ones are preserved, thus effectively halving the pulse rate.

   b. Alternation of the loudness of the second sound and of any ejection murmur may also be noted.

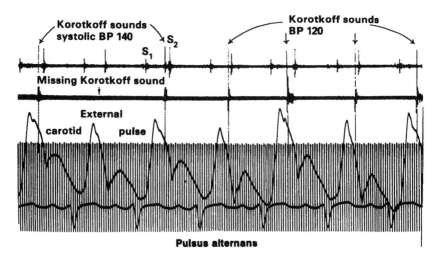

Pulsus alternans

The heart sounds are shown in the top line. The next line is taken with a microphone over the brachial artery distal to a blood pressure cuff. Note the doubling of the number of Korotkoff sounds when the cuff had been deflated from 140–120 mmHg.

4. Is pulsus alternans more or less likely with a high venous pressure? What is its significance?

    ANS: Less likely. Therefore it is more likely to be present with the legs dangling or after administration of a diuretic.

BLOOD PRESSURE AND PULSES IN THE LEGS _____

Normal Pressures

1. How does the blood pressure in the legs compare with that in the arms?

    ANS: With a proper-size cuff over the thigh, the popliteal systolic pressure should be either the same or as much as 20 mmHg higher than in the arms. If the systolic pressure in the legs is lower than that in the arms, occlusive disease anywhere beyond the origin of the subclavian arteries should be suspected.

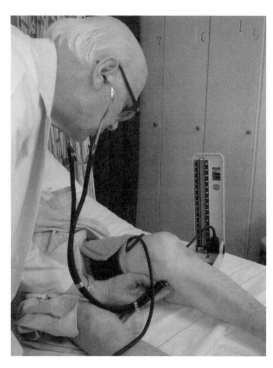

The usual commercial leg cuff, such as that shown here, must be rolled diagonally around the thigh, to keep the edges snug against the skin. The systolic blood pressure in the legs should not be over 20 mmHg higher than in the arms

2. Where is the most reliable place to auscultate for blood pressure in the legs?

    ANS: Over the popliteal artery with the large cuff on the thigh. (A bell chest piece is used.)

Note: Compressing the thigh with a blood pressure cuff can cause enough discomfort to cause a false elevation of pressure. When an accurate comparison with the brachials is necessary, as in patients with suspected coarctation or AR, the arm and thigh measurements should be done by two persons simultaneously.

3. How is the blood pressure taken in the lower legs?

   ANS: Place an arm cuff just above the malleolus (i.e., as close as possible to the posterior tibial artery) but without including the protuberance of the malleolus. Use a small (pediatric) bell to auscultate the posterior tibial artery. If no Korotkoff sounds are audible, auscultate or palpate the dorsalis pedis instead. If no Korotkoff sounds are present over any foot artery, the Doppler method can be used.

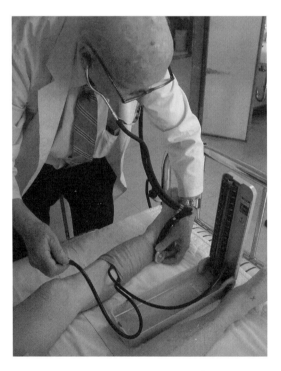

A convenient method of taking a leg pressure if you do not have a thigh cuff. A pediatric bell should be used to achieve an easy air seal behind the medical malleolus.

4. What are the disadvantages of using the foot rather than the thigh for taking a blood pressure?

   ANS: a. No Korotkoff sounds can be elicited over the posterior tibial or dorsalis pedis in about 10% of patients.

   b. Marked peripheral constriction, as in a cold room, may cause the
      blood pressure to be as much as 50 mmHg lower in the foot than in
      the arm.

5. How is blood pressure taken in an infant?

   ANS: a. By the flush method: the limb is raised until it is blanched (some
           bind the forearm with a bandage to empty it of blood first). Then the
           cuff is inflated. The first distal flush as the cuff is deflated is read as
           the mean pressure.
        b. By Doppler ultrasound: with a cuff about 2.5 cm wide, a systolic
           pressure can be obtained.

Leg Blood Pressure in Aortic Regurgitation

1. How does AR affect the blood pressure in the legs in comparison with that in the
   arms? What is this sign of AR called?

   ANS: AR exaggerates the tendency for the leg systolic pressure to be higher
        than that in the arms. If the difference is greater than normal, i.e., more
        than 20 mmHg, it is known as a positive Hill's sign [7].

   Note: It is easy to remember because blood pressure increases, i.e., goes
           "uphill" in AR as the examiner goes down the body.

2. Why is the cuff systolic pressure in AR higher in the legs than in the arms?

   ANS: One theory is that reflected waves from the periphery sum with for-
        ward waves. These summed waves are known as standing waves.

3. How can Hill's sign be used to grade the severity of AR?

   ANS: In mild AR the difference is up to 20 mmHg (i.e., the difference is in
        the normal range). In moderate AR the difference is 20–40 mmHg; in
        severe AR the difference is over 60 mmHg. A difference of between 40
        and 60 mmHg may represent either moderate or severe AR [8].

4. What produces a falsely low Hill's sign (i.e., less difference than would be
   expected from the severity of the AR)?

   ANS: a. Congestive heart failure, presumably because of the poor stroke
           volume. A positive Hill's sign may depend, at least in part, on a
           strong myocardial contraction.
        b. Significant AS.

Leg Pulses and Blood Pressure in Coarctation of the Aorta

1. When should you suspect coarctation of the aorta?

   ANS: In any patient with hypertension.

2. What are the characteristics of the pulses proximal to and beyond an aortic coarctation?

   ANS: The proximal pulses, i.e., the carotid and brachial pulses, are large, bounding pulses. The parts of the body beyond the coarctation (i.e., usually beyond the left subclavian artery) receive blood through enlarged collaterals that do not transmit the percussion wave well. Therefore, not only do the lower extremity pulses have a low pulse pressure, but also their rate of rise is slow and they have a late peak, i.e., the pulse wave is almost purely a tidal wave.

   Note: The blanching time (time required for normal color to return after firm pressure on the foot skin) is normally about 1.3 s in the toes, but averages over 3 s in the presence of coarctation.

3. If the onsets of the femoral and radial pulses are almost simultaneous, what causes the sensation of the delayed peak in the femorals?

   ANS: Because of the decreased initial flow rate through the femorals, their percussion wave is so low that only the tidal wave is felt in the femorals.

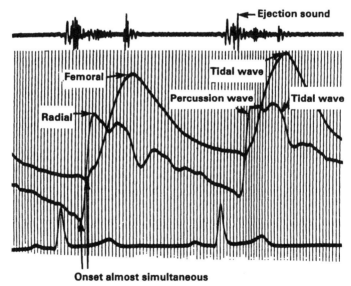

Onset almost simultaneous

Intra-arterial pressure tracings in a patient with coarctation of the aorta show that the onsets of the femoral and radial pulses remain almost simultaneous. In coarctation, a delay in the femoral is felt on palpating both arteries simultaneously because the percussion wave distal to an obstruction is obliterated by an anacrotic shoulder, which is imperceptible. Thus only the tidal wave is felt in the femoral artery, whereas the earlier percussion wave is felt in the unobstructed radial artery.

In the radials, the usual percussion wave is easily felt because there is no obstruction to flow.

4. How can you overcome the difficulties in timing and comparing the femoral and radial pulse peaks to look for a femoral delay?

ANS: a. Place the patient's wrist over the femoral artery, so that your fingers on the radial pulse are above your fingers on the femoral pulse.
b. Vary the compression force until both pulse pressures feel equal.
c. Femorals are best found with the legs slightly abducted and the foot externally rotated.

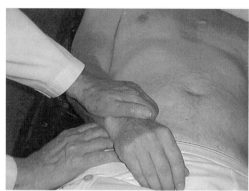

By placing the patient's wrist over his or her femoral artery as you palpate both, you can best perceive the obvious delay of the femoral pulse peak over that of the arm. In using the radials rather than the brachials to test for differences between the arm and leg, you take advantage of the increased rapidity of pulse rise as you palpate more peripherally down the arm.

5. When may the femoral pulse be surprisingly easy to palpate in coarctation and so make the test for femoral peak delay especially useful?

ANS: When coexistent AR is present (as may occur with a bicuspid aortic valve).

Note: a. As many as 50% of patients with coarctation may have a bicuspid aortic valve, which is commonly regurgitant.
b. Exercise will raise blood pressure to unexpectedly high levels in patients with coarctation.

PULSUS PARADOXUS

1. What is meant by pulsus paradoxus?

ANS: It is a marked fall in systolic blood pressure on inspiration.

2. Does the systolic blood pressure normally increase or decrease with inspiration? Why?

ANS: It decreases because:

a. Lung capacity increases with inspiration and the pulmonary vascular bed expands so that less blood moves from the lung into the left heart.

     b. Intrathoracic pressure decreases with inspiration. Because the aorta is an intrathoracic organ, its pressure will also drop.

3. Why did the term *paradoxus* come into use?

    ANS: A Kussmaul, in the late 1800s, originally described a marked drop in, or even loss of, blood pressure on inspiration in patients with constrictive pericarditis. He called it a "pulsus paradoxus," because he noticed that the apex beat did not change in any way, despite the loss of radial pulse with inspiration.

How to Elicit a Pathological Inspiratory Fall in Blood Pressure

1. With what depth of respiration is the test done?

    ANS: Not more than a moderate depth of respiration. You may tell the patient who breathes too shallowly to breathe "just a little more deeply, but not too deeply," only enough for you to see the chest movements easily out of the corner of your eye while watching the manometer.

2. On moderate inspiration and expiration, what is a positive paradoxus (i.e., how much blood pressure fall on inspiration is definitely abnormal)?

    ANS: A fall of 10 mmHg or more is generally agreed on in the literature. Experience, however, will show you that an inspiratory fall of about 6 mmHg is the upper limit of normal. Some of the probable reasons for believing that between 8 and 10 mmHg could be normal are errors such as the following:

      a. Subjects are asked to breathe too deeply or even to hold their breath on inspiration and expiration.

      b. The physician may fail to realize that as the cuff pressure is being lowered slowly below the level of the first Korotkoff sound on expiration, the blood pressure itself is often falling. Therefore, after hearing the Korotkoff sounds both on inspiration and expiration for the first time, the physician must reinflate the cuff to see if the systolic pressure has actually dropped while deflating the cuff.

      c. A fall of 5 mmHg could be a significant loss of systolic pressure and actually mean **tamponade** if the pulse pressure were markedly reduced, e.g., to 20 mmHg. (For example, if the blood pressure were 110/90, a 5-mmHg decrease with inspiration could occur with tamponade.)

3. Which patients have the greatest inspiratory fall in systolic pressures, those with constriction or those with tamponade?

    ANS: Only with tamponade are inspiratory drops of 20 mmHg or more found during quiet breathing. In chronic constrictive pericarditis, a pulsus paradoxus is actually uncommon unless it is subacute, with some fluid still present (effusive-constrictive).

Note: a. Effusive-constrictive means a combination of tamponade (fluid) and visceral pericardium constriction.

b. With deep inspiration, up to 15 mmHg may be lost.

Mechanism of Marked Inspiratory Fall of Blood Pressure

1. Why is there a more marked drop in stroke volume on inspiration in tamponade than in normals?

ANS: Because on inspiration left atrial pressure rises higher than pulmonary venous pressure and forward flow into the LV is attenuated or even stopped.

2. Why does tamponade cause the left atrial pressure to rise so high on inspiration that it impedes inflow from the pulmonary veins?

ANS: With inspiration the volume of the right ventricle (RV) is increased, stretching the pericardium and increasing intrapericardial pressure. This increased intrapericardial pressure is transmitted to the left atrium (which is covered with pericardium), and its pressure is also raised during inspiration.

Note: Septal bowing into the LV on inspiration also contributes to the decrease of LV volume on inspiration.

Causes of False Positive and False Negative Tests for Marked Inspiratory Fall in Blood Pressure

1. Why do some asthmatic patients seem to have a marked inspiratory fall in blood pressure?

ANS: Bronchospasm may raise the intrathoracic pressure very high (similar to a Valsalva maneuver), and inspiration will, by contrast, seem to lower the systolic pressure excessively. Actually, it is an expiratory rise in blood pressure, not an inspiratory fall.

2. When will there be no significant inspiratory fall in blood pressure despite marked tamponade?

ANS: a. If AR is present, the LV can fill from the aorta during inspiration.

b. In patients with a large atrial septal defect (ASD) the normal increase in systemic venous return to the RV on inspiration is almost balanced by a decrease in left-to-right shunt, so that the RV volume changes very little during inspiration.

c. If the LV diastolic pressure is very high.

CAPILLARY PULSATION

1. How do you elicit capillary pulsation (Quincke's sign)?

    ANS: Compress the skin of the face or hands with a glass slide, or exert slight pressure on the nail beds and watch for intermittent flushing. You can also transilluminate the nail bed with a flashlight against the pad of the patient's finger while shading the finger with the other hand.

2. What is the mechanism of capillary pulsations and what noncardiac conditions can cause it?

    ANS: The mechanism is the transmission of the arterial pulse through dilated capillaries to the subpapillary venous plexus. It is found in any condition that causes capillary dilatation, such as hot weather, a hot bath, fever, anemia, pregnancy, or hyperthyroidism.

3. Which cardiac conditions cause capillary pulsation?

    ANS: Any cardiac condition that causes a large pulse pressure, such as AR, systolic hypertension, or marked-bradycardia, as in complete **atrioventricular block**.

ABDOMINAL AORTIC ANEURYSM (AAA)

1. Which patients should be routinely screened for AAA?

    ANS: Patients with increased risk, especially those over age 50 with hypertension or coronary disease history.

2. How can palpation be used to screen for AAA?

    ANS: Note the separation of the index fingers with each systole with the hands placed on each side of the aorta. If the pulsating area is more than 2.5 cm in width after allowing for skin thickness, a pulsatile mass should be considered to be present. (Abdominal or femoral bruits are of no help.) In a thin abdomen, almost all AAA can be detected. On ultrasound, an AAA is a dilatation of more than 1.5 times the diameter of the proximal aorta.

HOW TO TELL CARDIAC FUNCTION BY BLOOD PRESSURE RESPONSE TO A VALSALVA MANEUVER

Normal Valsalva Hemodynamics

1. What happens to the blood pressure immediately on performing a Valsalva strain, and why?

    ANS: During the strain, the blood pressure rises by an amount equal to the increase in intrathoracic pressure because the aorta, like all structures in the thorax, must reflect changes in intrathoracic pressure.

2. What happens to the blood pressure, pulse pressure, and heart rate while the strain is maintained for 10 s?

    ANS: The blood pressure and pulse pressure decrease, and the heart rate increases. This occurs because the increased intrathoracic pressure obstructs venous return, and therefore progressively decreases stroke volume and cardiac output. The reflex sympathetic outflow due to the decreased stroke volume and blood pressure causes tachycardia.

3. What happens to the blood pressure, pulse rate, and heart rate on release of the strain?

    ANS: For a few beats the blood pressure falls owing to decreased flow into the LV, because there are a few seconds of decreased flow from relatively empty pulmonary vessels. Then the blood pressure overshoots to above control levels and the pulse pressure increases because the increased sympathetic outflow caused by the Valsalva maneuver persists for at least 5–10 s after the release of the strain and increases peripheral resistance. Added to this is the temporary increase in venous return to the heart of blood that had been dammed up by the increased intrathoracic pressure. This flow reaches the LV after a few seconds and causes an increase in LV stroke volume. The increased pressure on the carotid sinus, in turn, causes a reflex bradycardia.

The Valsalva Effect in Patients with Decreased Function

1. What is a normal ejection fraction?

    ANS: About $70 \pm 10\%$ of the end-diastolic volume that is ejected during systole by angiography.

2. What is the blood pressure response to a Valsalva strain if the ejection fraction is normal, i.e., $70 \pm 10\%$ by angiography, or $60 \pm 10\%$ by radionuclide methods?

    ANS: If the cuff pressure is held at 25 mmHg above systolic pressure during the strain, a few Korotkoff sounds heard at the beginning of the strain reflect the increased intrathoracic pressure. Then the Korotkoff sounds will disappear as the blood pressure falls, because of the decrease in venous return. Post-Valsalva, the Korotkoff sounds will reappear due to an overshoot of at least 25 mmHg if the ejection fraction is normal. If no overshoot is obtained, hold the cuff pressure at 15 mmHg above the control pressure. If there is an overshoot to 15 mmHg, the ejection fraction may be low normal or it may be slightly reduced.

3. What kind of blood pressure response to the Valsalva occurs with a markedly reduced ejection fraction?

    ANS: During the entire strain, the blood pressure stays up, and after the Valsalva maneuver there is no overshoot or bradycardia. This is known as

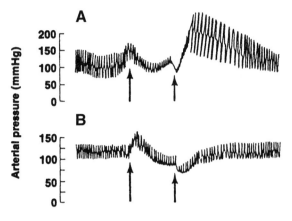

A. The typical normal blood pressure response to a 10-s Valsalva strain showing a good post-Valsalva overshoot, indicating an ejection fraction of about 70 ± 10%.

B. The absent post-Valsalva overshoot suggests an ejection fraction of about 50 ± 10% by angiography.

a *square-wave response*. This is partly due to the excess lung blood volume in the congested lungs, which continues to empty into the LV during the entire 10 s of strain.

4. How does the square-wave response relate to ejection fraction and end-diastolic pressure in the LV?

   ANS: It has been found that the ejection fraction is about 20 ± 10% by angiography (15 ± 10% by radionuclide methods). The end-diastolic pressure in the LV is likely to be very high (i.e., as much as 40 mmHg).

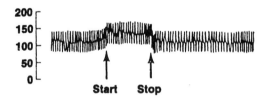

The square-wave response is present when there is no fall in blood pressure during and no rise in blood pressure after a Valsalva strain. This usually indicates an ejection fraction of 20 ± 10%.

5. What happens to the blood pressure response to the Valsalva if the ejection fraction is reduced to 50 ± 10% by angiography (40 ± 10% by nuclear methods) and has a near-normal ejection fraction only with the help of a high end-diastolic pressure?

   ANS: The blood pressure and pulse pressure decrease during the strain, but there is no poststrain overshoot [9]. This is presumably due to the excess sympathetic tone to which hearts with reduced ejection fractions are subject. Therefore, the strain does not stimulate enough further sympathetic drive to produce an overshoot after release of the strain.

6. What can produce a falsely abnormal absence of overshoot despite a normal heart?

    ANS: a. Any cause of autonomic imbalance, such as the use of beta blockers.
    b. Decreased blood volume.
    c. A moderate or large ASD.

    Note: A large ASD may even produce a square-wave response.

7. How can you help the patient to perform a Valsalva if he or she cannot comprehend your instructions or cooperate enough to carry out the maneuver?

    ANS: a. Press on the abdomen with one hand and ask the patient to push your hand away with the abdomen. If this does not work, then
    b. Have the patient blow up an aneroid manometer to 40 mmHg through a rubber tube connection. (A 20-gauge needle inserted into the rubber tube will ensure that continuous expiration through an open glottis is moving the manometer needle and prevents the needle from moving if only intra-oral pressure is raised.)
    c. Have the patient blow out hard against the resistance of the patient's forefinger inserted into his or her mouth.

    Note: Another way to use blood pressure to tell if the patient has low cardiac output is to divide the difference between systolic and diastolic blood pressure. This is known as the proportional pulse pressure. If the difference between systolic and diastolic blood pressure is 25% of the systolic pressure or less, then there is a 90% chance that the cardiac index is 2.2 L/min/m^2 or less.

REFERENCES

1. Corrigan, D. J. Permanent patency of the aortic valves. *Edinb. Med. Surg. J.* 37:225,1832.
2. Wood, P. Aortic stenosis. *Am. J. Cardiol.* 1:553,1958.
3. Harrison, E. G., Jr., Ruth, G. M., and Hines, E. A., Jr. Bilateral indirect and direct arterial pressures. *Circulation* 22:419,1960.
4. Rodbard, S., and Margolis, J. The auscultatory gap in arteriosclerotic heart disease. *Circulation* 15:850,1957.
5. Freis, E. D. Auscultatory indication of diastolic blood pressure. *Cardiol. Digest* 3:13, 1968.
6. Viol, G. W., et al. Seating as a variable in clinical blood pressure measurement. *Am. Heart J.* 98:913, 1970.
7. Hill, L., and Rowlands, R. A. Systolic blood pressure (1) in change of posture, (2) in cases of aortic regurgitation. *Heart* 3:219,1911–1912.

8. Frank, M. J., et al. The clinical evaluation of aortic regurgitation. *Arch. Intern. Med.* 116:357, 1965.
9. Zema, M. J., Caccavano, M., and Kligfeld, P. Detection of left ventricular dysfunction in ambulatory patients. *Am. J. Med.* 75:241,1983.

4 Jugular Pressure and Pulsations

VENOUS PRESSURE BY JUGULAR INSPECTION _____

1. With which chambers of the heart are the jugular veins in continuity in systole and in diastole?

    ANS: In systole the jugular veins are in continuity only with the right atrium, because the tricuspid valve is closed. In diastole, when the tricuspid valve is open, the jugulars are also in continuity with the right ventricle (RV). Therefore, examination of the jugulars may reveal the contour and pressure in the right atrium and RV without the need for catheterization.

In diastole, the atrium and ventricle are in continuity and become an "atrioventricle." Note also that the internal jugulars are in a more direct line with the superior vena cava than are the external jugulars.

Ventricular systole   Diastole

2. Why is the internal jugular a more accurate manometer than the externals?

    ANS: a. The internal jugulars are in a direct straight-line communication with the superior vena cave which, in turn, communicates directly with the right atrium. The external jugulars communicate with the superior vena cava after two near 90 turns, one where the external jugular enters the subclavian and another where the subclavian enters the superior vena cava. It is only logical that it would be difficult to communicate pressure accurately through two sharp turns.

b. The external jugulars are occasionally either absent or too thready to be visible to the naked eye in the normal population.

c. If the external jugulars are narrow in diameter under normal conditions, they become so constricted with heart failure or shock due to the increased sympathetic stimulation that they may become invisible.

3. When do internal jugulars become visible?

ANS: Only in the presence of severe tricuspid regurgitation.

4. If the internal jugulars are usually invisible, how can they be used as a manometer to measure venous pressure?

ANS: The pulsations of the internal jugulars are transmitted to the skin of the neck. The top level of the skin's pulsations is taken as the venous pressure. Thus the jugular is used as a "pulsation manometer."

5. Which is the most accurate internal jugular to use, the left or the right? Why?

ANS: Normally, the pressure in the right jugulars is either slightly greater than or the same as that in the left jugulars. Upper levels of normal have been established for the right side. In some arteriosclerotic patients the left jugular pressure may be falsely elevated owing to compression of the innominate vein between the sternum anteriorly and large tortuous arteries arising from a high unfolded aortic arch posteriorly. (An aortic **aneurysm** may also be the cause of innominate vein compression, but this is rare in comparison with arteriosclerotic compression.)

6. What does the expression, "The jugulars were (or were not) distended," imply?

ANS: This expression denotes several things:

a. The physician was using the external jugulars and therefore the absolute height of the venous pressure will be inaccurate. The external jugular top level of pulsations is usually lower than the top level of the internal jugulars.

b. When the statement is made that the jugulars were "flat" or "not distended," the internal jugular pulsations may still be very high if the external jugulars are either congenitally invisible or too constricted by the sympathetic stimulation of heart failure to be seen.

c. If the statement is made that the jugulars were distended to a high level with the chest elevated to 45 then you can probably believe that the venous pressure is actually high. This is because internal jugulars are almost always higher than external jugulars.

Boldface type indicates that the term is explained in the glossary.

7. When may you use external jugulars to measure venous pressure?

ANS: a. It is helpful to apply supraclavicular pressure with the chest elevated to 45 in an attempt to raise external jugulars when first looking at the neck for venous pressure. If the externals were invisible before supraclavicular pressure and can be distended by supraclavicular pressure, then they have a normal pressure and give a strong indication that the internal jugular pressures are also normal.

     b. In severe TR the RV systolic pressure transmits poorly to the external jugulars, which will more accurately reflect venous pressure.

HOW TO USE THE INTERNAL JUGULARS AS A MANOMETER ___

1. What reference level is used as zero?

ANS: The **sternal angle** (angle of Louis).

2. What are the upper limits of normal for jugular pulsation in the (a) supine and (b) 45 position with the sternal angle as zero?

ANS: a. The supine upper limit is 2 cm.

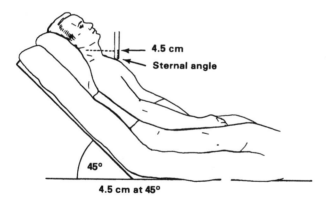

4.5 cm

Sternal angle

45°

4.5 cm at 45°

Venous pressure can be estimated by observing the upper level of internal jugular pulsations above the sternal angle. If it is over 4.5 cm at 45 , it indicates an

     b. The 45 upper limit is 4.5 cm. (It is easy to remember 4.5 cm at 45 .)

3. Why is it important to know the venous pressure at 45 rather than supine?

ANS: Supine, the top level of a normal venous pressure may not be seen because it could be above the angle of the jaw at mid-face level.

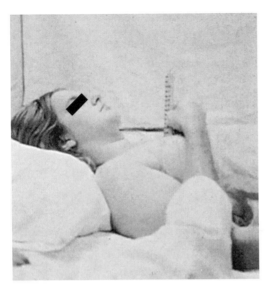

The 2-cm level is above the angle of the jaw in this patient. Therefore, only if her top level of pulsations were lower down at sternal-angle level would the upper level be measurable. At 45 , her top level of jugular pulsations was below jaw level and was measurable.

METHOD OF OBTAINING AN ACCURATE MEASUREMENT OF VENOUS PRESSURE

1. How can you detect jugular pulsations that are difficult to perceive?

    ANS: a. Shine a light tangentially from behind or in front of the neck to throw a jugular shadow.

    b. The most accurate way of finding the top level of pulsations is to examine the silhouette of the neck. When you are examining the right side of the neck, you must lean over to the left side of the patient or stand on the left side of the bed temporarily to obtain a good view of the silhouette of the skin overlying the right internal jugular.

    c. If the internal jugular pressure is high, the earlobes often pulsate. Unfortunately, a strong carotid pulse pressure can also cause slight earlobe pulsations.

2. What effect does inspiration have on jugular pulsations and their perception?

    ANS: The top level may be lower because the drop in intrathoracic pressure on inspiration may be reflected in the jugulars. Inspiration may, however, make jugular pulsations easier to see because the RV has more blood volume on inspiration and contracts with more energy.

    Note: Held respiration often eliminates jugular pulsations altogether, probably because of the slight Valsalva effect.

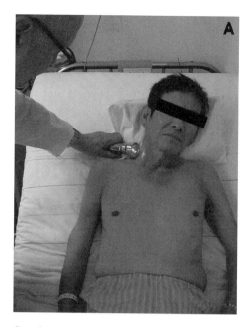
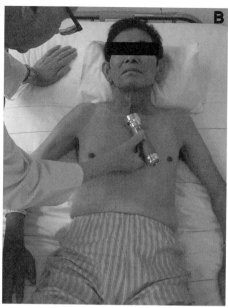

Jugular movements may be very subtle. Any slight movement of the hand holding the light can produce as much artifactual movement as movement from the jugulars themselves. Therefore, you must support your hand on either the pillow behind or the chest in front.

Leaning over to the left side of the patient to view an outline of the neck against the pillow will show you more subtle motion than could be seen even with an oblique light. Therefore, the true upper level of motion is best seen from this viewpoint.

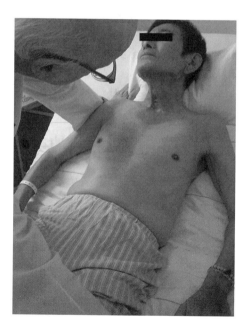

3. How can you obtain an accurate number in centimeters for a venous pressure?

ANS: Mark the upper level of jugular pulsation during inspiration with a felt-tipped pen. Place a tongue blade marked off in centimeters vertically on the **sternal angle**. The rounded ends make a tongue depressor the most comfortable measuring stick. A carpenter's level will give the most accurate vertical level. If no ruler is available, you may use the thickness of your fingers for a rough estimate. The second interphalangeal joint is generally about 2 cm in thickness. Measure your own joint for future use. If you place a closed fist on the sternal angle, each finger breadth is about 2 cm.

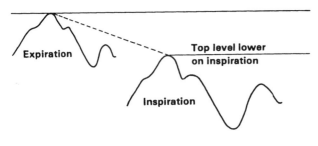

Note the higher absolute level but smaller amplitude of pulsations on expiration. With bronchospasm jugular pulsations with normal pressures may only be visible above the clavicle during expiration due to the effect of straining, which elevates intrathoracic pressure with each expiration.

HOW TO TELL JUGULAR FROM CAROTID PULSATIONS _____

1. How can you tell a jugular from a carotid pulsation by palpation?

ANS: Normal jugulars are not palpable. If the venous pressure is very high, you will occasionally feel an easily compressible, gentle undulation. The carotids produce a strong, almost incompressible impulse. Carotids are palpable as either a sharp tap if normal, or a push or nudge if there is aortic stenosis.

2. How can supraclavicular pressure help to separate jugular from carotid pulsations?

ANS: Since jugular pulsations arise from right atrial pulsations, supraclavicular pressure can eliminate jugular but never carotid pulsations. There is, however, a caution here. When internal jugular pulsations are very high and strong, they will not be eliminated by low supraclavicular compression. You must instead apply pressure at least halfway up the neck or even higher to eliminate these high-pressure jugular movements.

3. How can a sudden abdominal thrust help separate jugulars from carotids?

ANS: A sudden abdominal compression thrust will make the jugulars momentarily more visible but will have no effect on carotids.

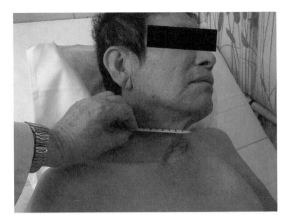

A very strong jugular pulsation with a high venous pressure will not be eliminated by pressure just above the clavicle, probably because the sternomastoid tendons prevent adequate pressure against the vein.

4. How can the contour of jugular movements help differentiate them from carotids?

   ANS: If the largest, fastest movement is inward, i.e., a collapse, then it is a jugular pulsation. The largest, fastest carotid movements are outward.

5. How does chest position help to distinguish jugulars from carotids?

   ANS: The more upright the chest, the lower the jugular pulsations are in relation to the clavicle because the right atrium becomes lower in relation to the clavicle in the upright position. The carotids, on the other hand, appear higher in the neck as the chest becomes more upright.

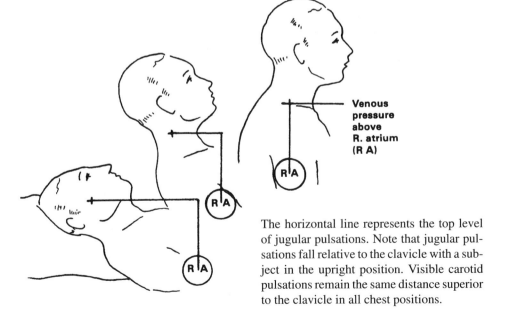

Venous pressure above R. atrium (R A)

The horizontal line represents the top level of jugular pulsations. Note that jugular pulsations fall relative to the clavicle with a subject in the upright position. Visible carotid pulsations remain the same distance superior to the clavicle in all chest positions.

THE ABDOMINAL COMPRESSION TEST (HEPATOJUGULAR REFLUX)

1. What is the cause of a high venous pressure in a person with low cardiac output?

    ANS: a. Increase of venous tone due to sympathetic outflow and catecholamines.

              b. Increased blood volume due to salt and water retention, probably at least partly due to the increased sympathetic outflow effect on the kidneys. One may therefore characterize a high venous pressure in heart failure as due to an increase in "tone volume."

2. What can cause a patient with heart failure to have an apparently normal venous pressure, despite an increase in tone volume, besides a diuretic?

    ANS: If a patient's normal venous pressure is 1 cm above the sternal angle at 45 , it may rise to only 3 cm; i.e., a 2-cm increase may occur when failure takes place. This is higher than normal for the patient but within normal limits for venous pressure.

3. What is the usual terminology for patients with congestive heart failure who have a high venous pressure and peripheral edema?

    ANS: Right ventricular (RV) failure.

4. What is unfortunate about the term RV failure?

    ANS: It has two meanings.

              a. Taken literally, it means that there is damage to the RV, as in RV infarction or inadequate ejection due to severe pressure overloads, as in severe pulmonary hypertension or stenosis.

              b. It is also used when there is a high venous pressure and peripheral edema even with intact RV function, as in patients with low output due to purely left ventricular problems. This latter is better given a different name, such as peripheral venous congestion.

5. How can you tell that a venous pressure below the upper limit of normal is actually high for that particular person?

    ANS: Abdominal compression will cause and maintain a rise in the top level of pulsations only if the venous pressure is relatively high. The greater the rise with abdominal compression, the higher the venous pressure. This is called *hepatojugular reflux* (not reflex).

6. What happens to the top level of jugular pulsations if abdominal compression is applied to a patient without heart failure? Why?

    ANS: The jugular venous pressure will fall because pressure on the abdomen obstructs femoral venous return almost as effectively as does venous tourniquets on the thighs. Thus, less blood reaches the right atrium.

Note: Abdominal compression that causes an increase in dyspnea or the use of accessory muscles of respiration implies that the patient's vital capacity is so reduced that he or she cannot tolerate any further decrease produced by pushing up on the diaphragm.

7. What is wrong with the historical term *hepatojugular reflux*?

   ANS: This term was first applied in 1885, when it was thought that pressure on a large liver was an essential part of the test and also that the procedure was a test only for tricuspid regurgitation. Actually, the effect can be achieved with a normal-sized liver and with compression on any part of the abdomen, although pressure on the right upper quadrant produces the greatest response. If the right upper quadrant is tender, do not hesitate to compress other areas instead. The term "hepatojugular reflux" has been retained because it is so widely known that it is useful for indexing and referencing as well as for communication among physicians.

   However, the term *positive abdominal compression* test is preferable when describing the results of abdominal pressure. The term *abdominal jugular test* has also been proposed, but for teaching purposes, the word *compression* is more specific.

   Note: A positive test has been correlated with a pulmonary capillary wedge pressure (left atrial pressure equivalent) of at least 15 mmHg.

8. Why does abdominal compression cause a sustained rise in pressure in a patient with congestive failure?

   ANS: The patient with peripheral venous congestion also commonly has a large RV and right atrium. Right upper quadrant compression transmitted to the RV and right atrium can interfere with their filling, especially if there is increased tone of those chambers and they are near the limit of their compliance. This may account for the fact that right upper quadrant pressure may cause a decrease in cardiac output, despite the apparently higher filling pressure.

9. What are the common causes of a false rise in the height of jugular pulsations with abdominal compression, i.e., not due to cardiac causes?

   ANS: a. Inability to tolerate the resistance to downward movement of the diaphragm when pressure on the abdomen raises the diaphragm in patients with severe obstructive pulmonary disease or in any other condition that causes severe loss of vital capacity.

   b. Increased blood volume, e.g., polycythemia vera.

   c. Increased sympathetic stimulation due to such causes as nervousness, pain, intravenous catecholamines, or an acute infarct.

Note: Abdominal compression often exaggerates the amplitude of the jugu-
        lar pulsations without actually raising the upper levels, and by merely
        revealing the true upper level of pulsations, which were difficult to
        perceive before compression, it may give a false impression of a rise
        in venous pressure.

10. How should you compress the abdomen in order to prevent false elevations due
    to sympathetic outflow?

    ANS: a. Compress with warm hands or with a garment or sheet between
             your hand and the abdomen.
          b. Spread the fingers apart, so that there is as little local pressure as
             possible.

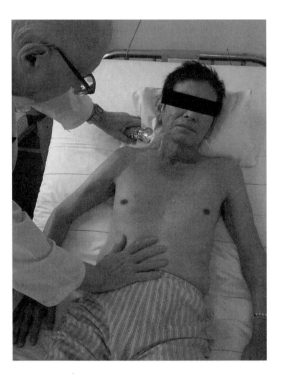

Spreading the fingers allows you to
distribute pressure over a large area, so
that more pressure can be applied without producing discomfort. Sometimes,
only marked abdominal pressure will
raise jugular pulsations enough to show
that they are abnormal.

          c. Start by pressing gently, and gradually increase the pressure to just
             below the point of discomfort.
          d. Ask the patient to tell you if you are pressing too hard, and warn
             him or her that it spoils the test if you produce discomfort.

11. What is Kussmaul's sign?

    ANS: Historically, Kussmaul's sign is the rise in the height of jugular pulsa-
          tions during inspiration in patients with chronic constrictive pericardi-
          tis. However, it is found in only a minority of patients with constrictive
          pericarditis, and it often occurs with peripheral venous congestion from
          any cause.

Note: a. Inspiration raises the intraabdominal pressures and can produce an
             effect like that of abdominal compression. Therefore, in any patient
             with a high venous pressure, inspiration may cause a further pres-
             sure increase.

         b. This sign should alert you to the presence of RV infarction in a
             patient with acute inferior infarction and no signs of left ventricular
             failure, because it will be present in a majority of such patients.

JUGULAR PULSE CONTOURS

Normal Jugular Pulse Contours

1. What is the difference between the jugular and right atrial pulse contours?

   ANS: None for all practical purposes, except when jugular pulse tracings pick
         up carotid artifacts. Therefore, the right atrial contours will be explained
         first because it is right atrial events that produce the jugular contours.

2. What is the normal right atrial contour and what are the letters given to the
   important crests and descents?

   ANS: The normal right atrial contours consist of A, C, V, and H waves. How-
         ever, it is also important to explain the descents, which should be called
         X, X prime (X′), and Y.

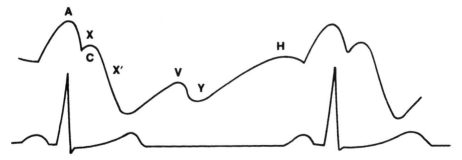

Right atrial pressure pulse waves. This is similar to what is recorded on a jugular pulse
tracing.

Radial pulse

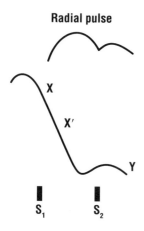

Because the X descent due to atrial relaxation is so small, the dominant descent during ventricular systole is the X′ descent.

3. What does the eye see on the neck of a normal adult? How does it differ from a jugular pulse tracing?

ANS: One systolic descent simultaneous with a radial pulse and falling on to the S_2. The C wave is not seen and the V wave and Y descent may be so small that they are not perceived. The systolic descent is mostly the X′ or descent of the base effect.

The A Wave, X Descent, C Wave, and X′ Descent

1. When the P wave of the ECG occurs, what atrial event results?

ANS: The right atrium contracts and produces a rise in right atrial pressures. Rises in atrial pressure are not named. When the right atrium relaxes, the right atrial pressure falls. The fall in pressure, when it is named, is called the X descent. (Not all cardiology texts give this descent a name [1].) The rise and fall produces a wave universally known as the A wave.

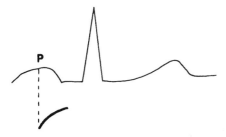

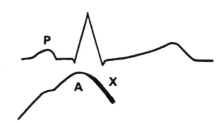

On the right atrial pressure curve, the rise in pressure resulting from atrial depolarization is not named.

Atrial relaxation produces the drop in pressure known as the X descent.

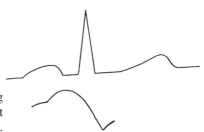

The rise in right atrial pressure due to bulging upward of the tricuspid valves into the right atrium has no name because it is not yet a wave.

2. What atrial event is initiated by the QRS?

    ANS: The QRS results in RV contraction that pushes up the tricuspid valve and raises the right atrial pressure slightly. This slight rise in pressure is not named.

3. Does the RV contract by approximation of its free wall to the septum, i.e., by movement of these structures toward each other? Does the apex move up toward the base?

    ANS: During systole the septum does not move toward the free wall of the RV and the apex does not move up. Normal RV ejection is due to two movements: The base moves downward and the free wall moves inward toward the septum.

    Note: Left ventricular (LV) ejection differs from RV ejection in that the septum and free wall move toward each other and the apex moves up slightly. In the RV the septum and free wall move in the same direction so that the RV depends much more on the descent of the base and the inward movement of the free wall.

The broken lines represent the four possible inward movements of the RV that could eject its blood. Only 1 and 4 occur normally.

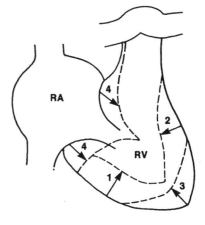

4. What happens to right atrial pressure when the floor of the atrium (base of ventricle) is pulled down during RV systole?

   ANS: Its pressure falls. This produces the major movement of the jugular pulse known as the X' descent. (This also produces a small wave known as the C wave.)

   Note: Only a minority of cardiologists name this descent, and most of those who do name it call it X, i.e., they give it the same name as that given to atrial relaxation, thus leading to great confusion [1].

The V Wave and Y Descent

1. When does RV contraction become too weak to continue pulling down the base? How does this affect right atrial pressure?

   ANS: The phase of reduced ejection occurs in mid-systole. This attenuates the descent of the base and allows the filling of the right atrium from the venae cavae to raise right atrial pressure. This rise in pressure during systole is not named.

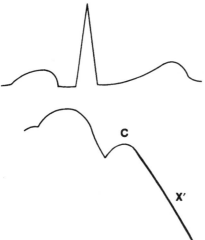

The C wave and X' descent. Most authors use the letter X to name both atrial relaxation and the fall in pressure due to the descent of the base, thus making the physiology of jugular contours difficult to understand.

2. What ends the rise in right atrial pressure and then allows the pressure to fall, thus making a wave?

   ANS: Right ventricular relaxation allows RV pressure to fall below right atrial pressure, thus opening the tricuspid valve (at the end of isovolumic relaxation).

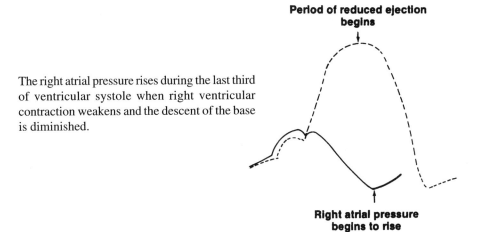

The right atrial pressure rises during the last third of ventricular systole when right ventricular contraction weakens and the descent of the base is diminished.

The atrial (and jugular) V wave is built up during systole while the tricuspid valve is closed.

3. What name is given to the wave and the descent produced by filling of the right atrium during ventricular systole followed by diastolic emptying?

   ANS: The V wave and Y descent.

4. Is the Y descent rapid or slow? Why?

   ANS: Rapid. It reflects the rapid expansion phase of the RV.

5. What is meant by saying that an "atrioventricle" results from opening of the tricuspid valve?

   ANS: When the tricuspid valve is open, the right atrium and ventricle form a common pressure chamber.

6. What happens to RV expansion after the end of the Y descent?

   ANS: A slow mid- and late-diastolic expansion phase occurs and the pressure in the atrioventricle rises slowly as blood pours into the RV. The wave so produced is called the H wave.

   Note: It is crucial to remember that the V wave is a systolic event occurring while the tricuspid valve is closed. It may help the novice to call the V wave a "villing" wave, i.e., a right atrial *filling* wave.

7. What name is given to the nadirs at the bottom of the X and Y descents? What is their significance?

   ANS: They are the X and Y troughs. They have no significance except that some textbooks, unfortunately, do not name descents at all but simply give the letters X and Y to the troughs.

Contour Recognition

1. Can you see a C wave by inspection of jugular neck pulsations?

   ANS: No. It is too small. The large C wave in jugular pulse tracings is due to carotid artifact because the pulse wave sensor that is used to record jugulars cannot separate out the impulse of a carotid movement, which occurs at about the same time as the tricuspid valve closure C wave. The C wave was originally thought to be entirely due to the carotid pulse, and thus the letter "C" for "carotid."

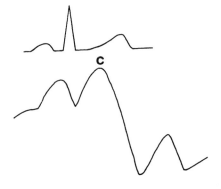

This jugular pulse tracing shows a large C wave that cannot be seen with the naked eye because it is due mostly to carotid artifact.

2. Why are the V wave and Y descent often not visible or very low in amplitude in most adults?

   ANS: Because the right atrium is a very compliant or distensible chamber, i.e., the right atrium is too distensible to allow its pressure to rise very much when the tricuspid valve is closed.

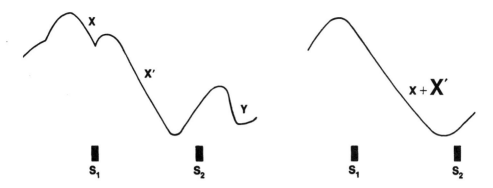

On the left is a normal jugular pulse tracing. On the right is the jugular pulse usually seen by the naked eye in the normal adult, i.e., one descent, the X plus X' but mainly the X'.

3. If a C wave, V wave, and Y descent are not seen in most adults, what should you look for on an adult jugular?

    ANS: You should expect to see a single systolic descent consisting only of a small X plus a large X'.

How to Time Normal Jugulars

1. Why is it easier to decipher jugular movements by observing descents or inward collapsing movements rather than ascents or outward movements?

    ANS: The jugular descents, or collapsing movements, are usually larger and faster than the ascents because the X' descent is due to RV contraction, which is rapid, and the Y descent is due to the rapid phase of RV expansion.

2. How can you recognize a dominant X' descent vs a Y descent by auscultation?

    ANS: Because the descent of the base, which causes the X' descent, is a systolic event, it must end at the end of systole, which is marked by the second heart sound (S_2). With your stethoscope, you can time the dominant jugular descent or collapse to see if it appears to fall onto the S_2. If it does, it is a dominant X', and the wave preceding it must be an A wave if the patient is in sinus rhythm. If, on the other hand, the dominant descent does not fall onto the S_2, it must be a Y descent, and the preceding wave must be a V wave (see figure above).

    Note: If there is an X' descent but very little Y, you may say that a dominant A wave is present if the patient is in sinus rhythm. This is a normal contour. If the Y is larger than the X', then a dominant V wave is present, which is always abnormal.

3. How can you time jugular descents by palpating peripheral pulses?

   ANS: Since both the radial pulse and the X′ descent are systolic, they bear a close temporal relationship to each other. The radial pulse occurs simultaneously with the X′ descent.

   Note: A carotid pulse occurs slightly before the jugular systolic collapse.

4. How does the jugular pulse in a young person differ from that in an adult?

   ANS: It is normal for the Y descent to be easier to see in a young person than in an adult because the **circulation time** is slightly faster in young people than in adults and the child's right atrium is relatively small for the volume it receives. This tends to raise a higher pressure in the right atrium and make a slightly larger V wave and Y descent in children than in adults.

Making the Jugular Pulsations Easier to See

1. Which jugulars should you examine for contours, the internal or the external jugulars? Why?

   ANS: Because they have the freest communication with the right atrium the internals are best. Occasionally, however, the external jugulars show the only easily analyzable movement.

2. Why should you place the patient in the supine position to examine for jugular contours?

   ANS: In the supine position, more blood returns to the right atrium. Furthermore, when the chest is raised, the jugulars may disappear below the clavicles.

3. How can you exaggerate jugular movement that is too small to be easily timed?

   ANS: Try to increase the venous return by elevating the subject's legs and having the subject take deeper breaths. Deep inspiration can draw more blood into the right atrium, making movements of larger amplitude.

   Note: a. The position for seeing the greatest magnitude of venous pulsation may vary from horizontal to upright, the latter in patients with very high venous pressure.

   b. Waveforms of the internal jugular vein are sometimes more easily perceived if the patient is rotated to about 50–75 , with the trunk at 30–45 .

Summary of Differences between Jugular and Carotid Pulsations

1. The carotid pulse has only one descent, or collapse; the jugular often has two, the X′ and the Y.

2. The carotid descent is slow, whereas the jugular X′ descent is rapid. If the fastest and greatest movement is a collapse, or descent, it is a jugular pulse.

3. Firm pressure just above the clavicle will obliterate all but the highest pressure jugular pulsations but will not affect carotid pulsations.

4. Inspiration may exaggerate jugular pulsations but will, if anything, diminish carotid pulsations.

5. Sitting up will make the carotids appear higher in the neck, but the jugulars will appear lower in the neck.

6. The carotid, if visible, is always easily palpable with firm pressure. The normal jugular is rarely palpable, except as a slight fluttering sensation with light pressure. The jugular is relatively easily compressible.

7. The X′ descent ends at the S_2, whereas the carotid descent appears to begin with the S_2.

8. Sudden abdominal compression makes the jugulars momentarily more visible but has no effect on the carotids.

Summary of How to Recognize Normal Jugulars

1. With the patient supine, palpate the radial pulse. If the jugular descent occurs simultaneously with the radial pulse, a dominant X′ descent is present.

2. Listen to the heart sounds and time the descents. If the nadir (bottom) of the descent falls onto the S_2, the dominant descent is an X′.

3. If you are still uncertain because of an irregular rhythm, you can confirm your impression by looking at the peaks of the jugular outward movements. If the dominant peak is simultaneous with the S_1, there is a dominant A wave, which is one of the characteristics of a normal contour. If simultaneous with the S_2, there is a dominant V wave.

Abnormal Jugular Contours

The Giant A Wave

1. How high is abnormally high for an A wave?

   ANS: Over 4.5 cm above the sternal angle with the chest at 45 .

2. What is an A wave called if it is higher than normal due to too strong an atrial contraction?

   ANS: A giant A wave.

   Note: a. A stronger-than-normal right atrial contraction may not produce a giant A wave but only a jugular "flicker" in the right supraclavicular area.

   b. A loud "knocking" sound accentuated by inspiration may be heard
      in the neck in the presence of a giant A wave.
3. What can cause an exaggerated atrial contraction?
   ANS: a. Obstruction at the tricuspid valve due to either tricuspid stenosis or
            right atrial tumor, such as a right **atrial myxoma**.
         b. A noncompliant or stiff RV due to either pulmonary outflow obstruc-
            tion, as with pulmonary stenosis, or pulmonary hypertension.
   Note: The right atrium contracts strongly when the tricuspid valve is obstructed
            because the atrium is stretched by the increased residual volume pro-
            duced by its inability to empty adequately through the obstructed orifice.
4. Why does an RV systolic pressure overload as in pulmonary stenosis or pulmonary hypertension cause a stronger than normal atrial contraction?
   ANS: When the RV has a pressure load to overcome, it becomes thicker and
         less compliant than normal. Because in diastole the atrium and ven-
         tricle are in continuity, the pressure in this atrioventricle rises very rap-
         idly as it fills with blood. The stretch of the atrium produces a **Starling
         effect** and a powerful atrial contraction which, in turn, stretches the
         ventricle before it contracts. The Starling effect on the ventricle strength-
         ens its contraction.

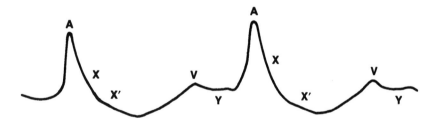

Tricuspid stenosis—This jugular pulse tracing from a patient with tricuspid stenosis shows a very slow Y descent due to difficulty in emptying the right atrium in
diastole. The X' descent (descent of the base) is also slow, probably because of
a poor right ventricular contraction caused by an underfilled right ventricle. Clinically, you could see that this patient had a giant A wave because the top level of
the jugular pulsation was high. It was 6 cm from the sternal angle with the chest
at 45 elevation (upper normal is 4.5 cm).

The Cannon Wave

1. What is a cannon wave?
   ANS: It is the high A wave caused by atrial contraction against a closed tri-
         cuspid valve.

2. When will the atrium contract against a closed tricuspid valve?

    ANS: When there is **atrioventricular dissociation** or when a very early P
    wave occurs on a T wave, as with a premature atrial contraction or a
    junctional pacemaker.

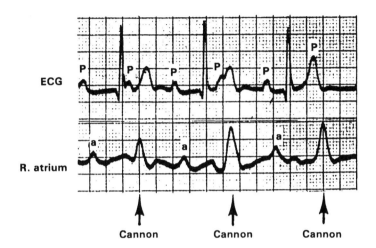

    Note that in this patient with complete atrioventricular block, every
    other P wave happens to fall on a T wave, i.e., it occurs during
    ventricular systole when the tricuspid valve is closed. Thus, there is
    a cannon A wave with every other P wave.

3. Are cannon waves easy or difficult to see?

    ANS: Cannon waves are usually very difficult to see unless the atrial contrac-
    tion is very strong, as when there is increased stiffness of the RV, such
    as in pulmonary hypertension. Because they are easily recorded, they
    were probably given the name cannon waves from the appearance on
    pulse tracings rather than from the appearance of the slight variations
    in jugular pulsation seen in the neck.

Abnormalities of the X' Descent

1. What are the usual conditions that can attenuate the X' descent?

    ANS: a. A poor RV contraction, as in RV infarction, or when there is no
        atrial presystolic Starling effect stretch, as in atrial fibrillation or
        flutter.
        b. Tricuspid regurgitation (TR), because the X' descent is encroached
        upon in proportion to the degree of regurgitation.

2. What can increase the amplitude of the X′ descent?

    ANS: a. Increased volume in the RV, as with an atrial septal defect (ASD), pulmonary regurgitation, and **anomalous pulmonary venous connection**.

          b. Pericardial tamponade. Filling is restricted throughout diastole so that blood can only enter the right atrium during systole to make a good X′ descent. The slow filling during diastole may eliminate the Y descent.

Abnormalities of the V Wave

1. How can you recognize a higher than normal V wave at a glance?

    ANS: By recognizing a Y descent of greater amplitude than normal.

2. What are the common causes of a higher than normal jugular V wave?

    ANS: a. Excessive right atrial filling either from (1) above the tricuspid valve, as in ASD or anomalous pulmonary venous connection, or (2) below the tricuspid valve as in TR.

          b. Loss of **compliance** of the right atrium from either (1) outside the heart, i.e., constrictive pericarditis, or (2) inside the heart, i.e., atrial tumors or high diastolic pressures in the atrioventricle due to the RV hypertrophy of pulmonary outflow obstruction or heart failure.

3. How does the high V wave of excess right atrial filling from above the tricuspid valve (e.g., ASD) differ from the V wave of TR?

    ANS: In ASD there is a large X′, as well as a large Y descent giving a prominent double descent. The large X′ is due to the large volume ejected by the RV pulling vigorously down on the floor of the atrium. In TR the regurgitant wave tends to obliterate the X′ descent.

4. Why is it easy to distinguish the prominent double descent of uncomplicated ASD from that due to constrictive pericarditis?

    ANS: In constrictive pericarditis the venous pressure will be elevated above normal and usually a Y descent is dominant. Constrictive pericarditis produces an early diastolic dip and plateau, i.e., an exaggerated Y ending with an abrupt jerky rise (Friedreich's sign). In uncomplicated ASD the venous pressure is normal and the X′ is usually dominant.

    Note: In restrictive cardiomyopathy the jugular pressure and waves are similar to that of constrictive pericarditis, i.e., the jugular pressure is elevated and may have an X′ with a dominant Y descent.

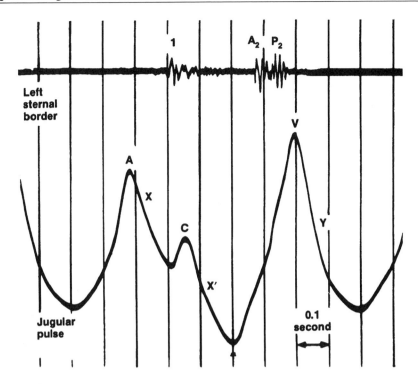

Shown is a jugular pulse tracing from patient with an atrial septa defect since the eye cannot see the C wave, it appears to be only a large double descent with the systolic descent (X plus X') appearing larger than the Y descent.

As the degree of TR increases, the X' descent is increasingly encroached upon. With severe TR, no X' descent is seen, and the jugular pulse is said to be "ventricularized."

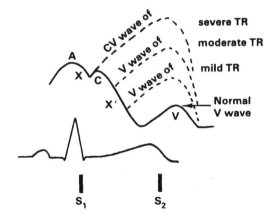

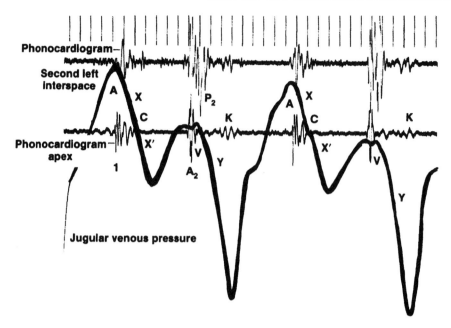

Severe constrictive pericarditis. Shown is a jugular pulse tracing from a patient with severe constrictive pericarditis. Note the double descent with a dominant Y descent and relatively small X′ descent. K indicates a pericardial knock sound. (From E. Craige, Heart Sounds. In E. Braunwald [ed.], *Heart Disease* [2nd ed.]. Philadelphia: Saunders, 1984).

5. Why does cardiac surgery usually result in an increase in Y descent at the expense of the X′ [2]?

    ANS: a. Sutures in the right atrium to close the opening made for tube insertion can cause loss of compliance of the right atrium.

    b. The right atrial pericardium may not be suspended firmly to the surrounding structures after surgery so that when the floor of the atrium is pulled down by RV contraction the entire atrium tends to move down more than normally, i.e., the atrial resistance to a downward pull is attenuated.

6. Why will a high mid-diastolic pressure of pulmonary hypertension or stenosis have a high V wave?

    ANS: Pulmonary hypertension or stenosis thickens the RV, thus raising the diastolic pressures. If there is a high pressure in this common atrioventricular (AV) chamber throughout diastole, then when the tricuspid valve is closed during systole the atrial V wave rises from a baseline that is higher than normal.

Summary of Jugulars in Tamponade and Constrictive Pericarditis

In tamponade:	A dominant X' descent and almost absent Y.
In constriction:	A dominant Y descent with a rebound wave after the Y trough and with a small X'.
In effusive constrictive or mild constrictive pericarditis:	A dominant X' with a fair Y almost equal to the X'.

The Jugulars in Atrial Fibrillation (AF)

1. Why will AF attenuate the X' descent and cause a dominant Y descent?

    ANS: In AF the RV contraction is decreased due to a lack of a booster pump effect of atrial contraction at the end of diastole.

2. Why will a patient in AF with congestive heart failure often have no X' descent at all, i.e., only a Y descent may be seen?

    ANS: a. The decrease in RV contraction due to the decreased venous return causes a decreased descent of the base.

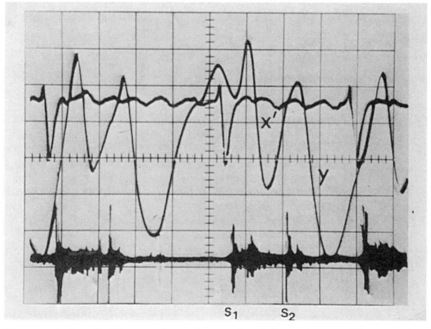

The wave before the X' cannot be an A wave since it is not due to atrial contraction. Note the good X' descent, despite the dominant Y descent, in this patient with moderate rheumatic MR.

   b. The right atrium in a patient with heart failure is under increased
      tension from excess sympathetic stimulation and from the high pres-
      sure in the atrioventricle when the AV valve is open. Thus the atrium
      is less compliant than normal. Therefore, there will be a steeper rise
      in atrial pressure as it receives its blood from the venae cavae to
      build up a V wave during ventricular systole.

3. What is the name of the wave preceding the X′ in AF?

   ANS: An H wave.

4. How can you quickly tell that the major descent that you are seeing is a Y descent
   in the presence of rapid AF?

   ANS: Auscultation is the best method for rapid rates. At rapid rates a Y descent
        falls onto the S_1. With rapid rates you may also make use of peaks as well
        as descents because with an X′ descent, the peak of the jugular move-
        ments occur with the S_1. With AF the peak is reached at the time of the S_2.

REFERENCES

1. Constant, J. The X prime descent in jugular contour nomenclature and recognition.
   Am. Heart J. 88:372, 1974.
2. Matsuhisa, M., et al. Postoperative changes of jugular pulse tracing. *J. Cardiogr.*
   6:403, 1976.

5

Inspection and Palpation of the Chest

VENTRICULAR ENLARGEMENT FROM EXAMINATION OF THE CHEST

Terminology Problems

1. What is the difference between cardiac enlargement and cardiac hypertrophy?

   ANS: Cardiac enlargement means dilatation or increase in chamber volume with or without proportionate hypertrophy, i.e., not hypertrophy alone. Pure hypertrophy should not be called enlargement because the chamber volume may remain normal or even be encroached on by the hypertrophied muscle.

2. What is usually meant by the term *apex beat*?

   ANS: It refers to the apex of the left ventricle (LV).

3. How does the apex of the LV actually relate to the apex beat?

   ANS: The part of the heart striking the chest wall is not necessarily the LV apex. In patients with a large enough right ventricle (RV), the apex beat may be due to an RV impulse.

4. What two forces produce the usual palpable LV apex beat?

   ANS: During isovolumic contraction, the heart rotates counterclockwise as viewed from below and usually the lower part of the anterior LV strikes the chest wall. Also, a recoil force produced by the ejection of blood into the aorta in an upward, rightward, and posterior direction thrusts the LV against the chest wall in an inferior, leftward, and anterior direction, a thrust opposed by the systolic decrease in cardiac volume.

5. What is meant by the term *PMI*, and what are the term's drawbacks?

   ANS: The term PMI is often used as a synonym for an apex beat. However, it has also been used to mean *point of maximum intensity*, i.e., the site of the loudest murmur. Second, as stated in the pamphlet prepared by Hurst and Schlant for the Committee on Medical Education for the American Heart Association, the term PMI should be avoided because the maximum precordial pulsations may be due to such abnormalities as a dilated pulmonary artery, a large RV, a ventricular **aneurysm**, or an aortic aneurysm. In describing what is thought to be the most lateral cardiac impulse nearest the true apex, the preferable term, even though not perfect, is apex beat.

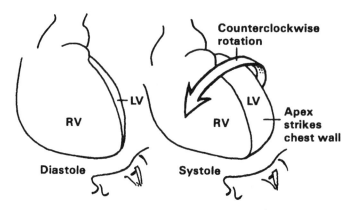

This counterclockwise rotation occurs during isovolumic contraction, i.e., before blood is ejected from the ventricles.

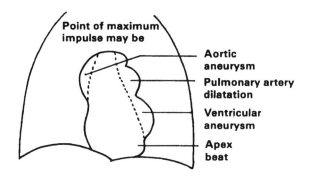

The point of maximum impulse (PMI) should not be equated with the apical impulse.

Note: Palpate around the right sternoclavian joint for the faint pulsations of a right-sided aortic arch, which is common in severe tetralogy or pulmonary atresia. Also palpate the sternal area for the pulsation of a large aneurysm of the descending aorta pushing the heart forward during systole.

Boldface type indicates that the term is explained in the glossary.

Chest Position to Find the Apex Beat

1. Why is the sitting position with the feet on the bed the best position to establish the site of the normal apex beat?

    ANS: It is the most compatible compromise with the familiar normal apex site on a chest X-ray. Also, in the sitting position the apex beat often becomes more palpable than it does even standing, because with the legs on the bed the upward compression by the abdominal contents and diaphragm shifts the apex beat slightly to the left against the chest wall.

2. Does the apex beat move laterally or medially when going from standing to sitting?

    ANS: The sitting position probably does not shift the apex beat laterally any more than 1 cm compared to the usual standing X-ray.

Palpability of the Apex Beat

1. About how often can you expect to feel an apex beat in normal subjects over age 40?

    ANS: Only in about one out of five [1]. However, in about 90% of children and teenagers, an apex beat is palpable in the sitting position. An apex beat is much more likely to be palpable in the sitting than in the supine position because in the latter, the heart falls away from the anterior chest wall. In the **left lateral decubitus position**, however, the apex beat may be palpable in about four out of five older adults, and in most children and young adults. It may require elevation of the chest to about 30 and various degrees of left lateral rotation in order to palpate a subtle apex beat.

2. How does obesity or a thick chest affect palpability of an apex beat? Their significance?

    ANS: A thick chest in an obese young person does not necessarily make the normal LV impulse impalpable, probably because the heart is physiologically enlarged in obesity. However, if the chest wall is thick and the posteroanterior diameter is increased in a patient over age 50, the mere palpability of an apex impulse may be used as a sign of cardiomegaly.

3. What unusual approach may sometimes help you to feel a subtle apex beat or an unexpectedly posterior axillary line apex beat?

    ANS: You should establish a routine of palpation from behind as well as from the front. A subtle apex beat may only be perceived when the hand palpates from a quiet immobile area like the back. The anterior chest is often disturbed by left parasternal movements and heart sound vibrations. Also, a frontal approach alone might mislead you into thinking that the movement you palpate on the anterior chest wall is the most lateral impulse when, in fact, it may be only an RV movement or an aneurysm, and the true LV apex beat may be missed because it may be near the posterior axillary line.

Note: When examining for an apex beat on a new patient, also palpate the right anterior chest (in the sitting position) so as not to miss a diagnosis of dextrocardia.

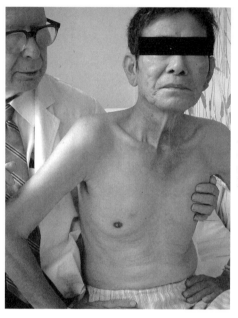

A posterior in addition to an anterior approach may allow you to feel more subtle movements, especially if your left hand is more sensitive than your right.

4. During what phase of respiration is the apex beat most palpable?

    ANS: The apex beat may come out between the ribs during any phase of respiration.

5. Which part of the hand is best for feeling the faint localized movement of a subtle apex beat? The right hand or the left hand?

    ANS: The fingertips or the area just proximal to them seems best for feeling a faint localized movement. Try each hand separately. Some examiners find that the fingers of one hand, usually the left in right-handed physicians, are more sensitive than the fingers of the other hand.

    Note: It is easy to mistake the vibrations of the first sound for a slight impulse, especially if it is not appreciated that heart sounds may be palpable.

The Normal Site of an Apex Beat

1. What is the disadvantage of using the midclavicular line as the site of the normal apex beat in the sitting position (with the feet on the bed)?

    ANS: a. Some medical dictionaries equate the midclavicular line with the nipple line to which it may bear no relation.

    b. The lateral end of the clavicle is often difficult to locate accurately.

2. What is an easier, more accurate method of finding the site of an apex beat in order to diagnose cardiomegaly?

    ANS: With the patient sitting up in bed with the legs on the bed, measure from the midline of the chest to the site of the apex beat. The normal apex beat is not more than 10 cm from the midline. However if you wish to predict what the X-ray will show, you must measure from the midline to the most lateral cardiac impulse and not to the point of maximum impulse (PMI).

    Note: a. The upright position of the chest to locate a cardiac impulse is superior to the supine position because it brings the heart closer to the chest wall. In the supine position the heart falls away from the chest wall.

    b. An upright position is more like a chest X-ray position. This is more logical than a supine position if you are trying to predict what the standing X-ray will show.

3. Why is it useless to estimate the site of the apex beat in the left lateral decubitus position?

    ANS: Variations in mediastinal mobility make the determination of a normal apex beat site in the left lateral position valueless.

4. Why is it usually of no clinical value to record the rib interspace in which the apex impulse is palpable?

    ANS: This is because the ribs curve downward as they sweep forward from behind so that the fifth interspace at the anterior axillary line is at a higher horizontal level than is the fifth interspace at the parasternal line.

    Note: A **pectus excavatum** and congenital complete absence of the pericardium can displace an LV impulse to the left in the absence of cardiomegaly [2].

5. Why is chest percussion for cardiac size not employed by most cardiologists?

    ANS: a. A palpable ventricular apical impulse indicates the heart size quickly. When a ventricular impulse is not palpable because of a thick chest or overaeration due to pulmonary disease, percussion is most unreliable, i.e., when percussion is most needed, it is of least help.

    b. Dressler, who devoted 20 pages of his textbook on clinical cardiology to percussion, begins by stating that he finds it impossible to percuss cardiac borders [3]. His 20 pages are devoted to a system for defining areas of cardiac dullness, which gave him information concerning specific chamber enlargement.

CARDIAC DILATATION SIGNS
IN THE LEFT LATERAL DECUBITUS POSITION

1. With the patient in the left lateral decubitus position, how can you tell that you are feeling a left or right ventricular apical impulse?

    ANS: There are two methods.

        a. Palpate the apical impulse to see if there is a sensation of a localized thrust. In the left lateral decubitus position an LV impulse feels as if a Ping-Pong ball were protruding between the ribs in systole. An RV impulse is usually more diffuse.

        b. Look for medial or lateral retraction. An LV impulse will manifest medial retraction because the counter-clockwise rotation of the heart causes a decrease in volume of the RV and outflow tract during systole, which causes the medial aspect of the heart to withdraw from the chest wall and pull on any overlying chest wall structures including the skin. The skin movement is often too subtle to be detected by palpation and is best detected by observing the skin while palpating the apex beat. A mark on the skin made by a pen may aid in seeing slight medial retraction. An RV apical impulse will often show lateral retraction.

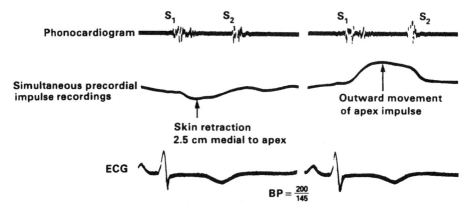

Note the retraction medial to the apex. The apex has a sustained impulse due to the effect of LVH. Although these tracings were taken in the supine position, medial retraction is best seen in the left lateral decubitus position.

2. How can you tell that there is cardiac enlargement with the patient in the left lateral decubitus position?

   ANS: Look for

   a. An enlarged area of apical impulse in the Y axis, i.e., an apical impulse should not be felt in more than one interspace.

   b. An enlarged area of apical impulse in the X axis, i.e., an apex impulse should be no more than 3 cm from side to side (about 1½ finger breadths).

The normal apex beat is not felt in two interspaces during the same phase of respiration.

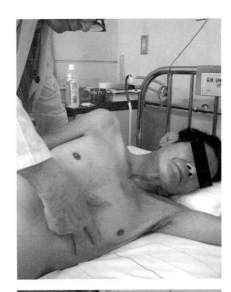

A normal apical impulse is no larger than about 1½ fingertip widths (3 cm).

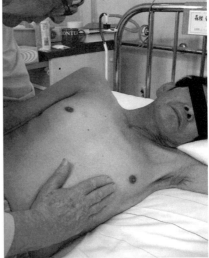

c. An enlarged area of medial retraction. The normal area of medial retraction is not much larger than that of the normal apex beat.

d. The presence of a combination of both medial and lateral retraction. If the medial retraction is dominant, you are probably feeling a large LV. If the lateral retraction is dominant, a large RV is probably producing the apical impulse.

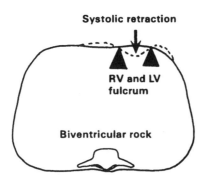

Retraction in the mid-left thorax, with sustained outward movements on either side, tells you that there is a biventricular volume overload.

e. A biventricular overload, as in a large ventricular septal defect (VSD) may be manifest on the chest wall as a biventricular rock, i.e., both the left parasternal and apical areas may rise with systole, with an area of retraction between them.

RIGHT VENTRICULAR ENLARGEMENT

1. How can you best palpate for movement caused by a large RV?

ANS: a. Since the RV is an anterior structure, its enlargement may produce an increased left parasternal movement. Diffuse left parasternal movements are often best palpated with the proximal part of the palm (thenar and hypothenar areas). The movement is then transmitted to the entire arm. The shoulder becomes the fulcrum and this amplifies the hand movements that are at the end of the arm lever.

b. Look for systolic downward movement in the epigastrium. If you place the pad of your right thumb pointing upward just beneath the xiphoid process, an impulse striking your thumb pad is usually due to a large RV. The downward impulse may be only palpable at the end of a deep, held inspiration.

Note: Occasionally the movement of a dilated pulmonary artery in the second left interspace imparts a movement to the overlying skin even though it is impalpable. Press firmly with one or two fingers over the second left interspace. Localized movements are best felt with the

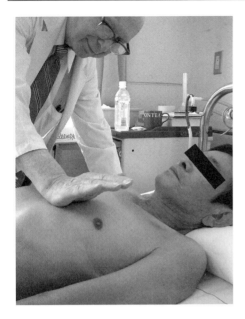

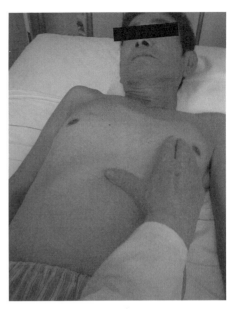

In this patient with mitral stenosis, the physician is palpating the movement of a large RV, which was producing a right ventricular rock, i.e., a sustained left parasternal impulse and lateral retraction.

If your fingernails are long enough to cause discomfort when you push up into the epigastrium with your fingers, you may use the pad of your thumb to test for RV pulsations during a deeply held inspiration.

tips of the fingers. The degree of pulmonary artery dilatation that will cause a visible or palpable movement is usually seen only with the dilated RV caused by severe primary pulmonary hypertension or by RV volume overloads, such as with **atrial septal defects**.

2. How can you diagnose the presence of a large RV in the left lateral decubitus position?

ANS: Look for dominant lateral retraction.

A sustained left parasternal impulse with lateral retraction is a sign of a volume overload of the RV (and probably also with the addition of a pressure overload).

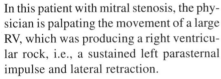

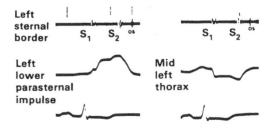

3. What causes the lateral retraction seen with RV enlargement due to severe tricuspid regurgitation (TR)?

    ANS: The lateral retraction seen with severe TR has been explained by two phenomena. First, there is an abnormally large inward movement of the apical region, which is formed by the dilated RV. Added to this is the simultaneous anterior thrust of the RV against the left parasternal area caused by the ballistic recoil response of the RV as it ejects its blood through the incompetent tricuspid valve.

4. How can severe TR affect the entire right and left precordium?

    ANS: If the TR is severe, the anterior left parasternal movement together with the apical retraction creates a rocking motion that has been called a right ventricular rock. Sometimes the entire right precordium may expand during systole due to the expanding right atrium, while the entire left precordium, including the parasternal area, retracts, probably because the RV, like an overdistended balloon in diastole, empties during systole and may draw in the entire left parasternal area and even the entire left chest.

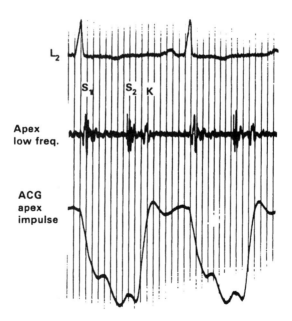

Apex cardiogram and phonocardiogram of a 25-year-old man with constrictive pericarditis due to uremic pericarditis and hemopericardium. Note the early S_3 or pericardial knock (K), the systolic apical retraction, and the diastolic outward movement.

5. When will the most lateral ventricular impulse retract deeply in systole without the initial outward movement that is seen in RV overload?

    ANS: In constrictive pericarditis. The apical retraction in systole is usually followed by a diastolic outthrust. The outward impulse at the apex is diastolic and not systolic as is seen with the usual apex beat.

6. What is the significance of a fixed anterior left chest bulge as seen from the foot of the bed?

    ANS: You should suspect an atrial septal defect with pulmonary hypertension, because the left chest bulge here is presumably due to the occurrence in infancy of a large shunt with hyperkinetic pulmonary hypertension. The large hyperactive and hypertrophied RV under high pressure can push the left chest forward as the skeleton is developing. The RV never enlarges to the right on chest X-rays, i.e., the right border of the heart with no congenital **malpositions** is never due to the RV, no matter how large it becomes. Therefore, RV enlargement does not affect the right anterior chest but instead will cause a left precordial bulge.

    Note: A systolic VSD shunt cannot enlarge the RV during systole, but a large shunt can increase end-diastolic volumes up to 2 1/2 times normal by shunting during isovolumic relaxation and also during diastole.

LEFT-SIDED CAUSES OF LEFT PARASTERNAL MOVEMENT _____

1. When is mid- to lower-left parasternal movement due to the LV?

    ANS: a. In young subjects with long, thin chests, the LV impulse may be very medial (i.e., at the left parasternal area).
    b. In some subjects in whom the LV is markedly enlarged, the movements may extend medially to the left parasternal area (as well as laterally).
    c. The movement may occur in the presence of a ventricular aneurysm, in which case it will be sustained with a late peak.

2. When is the left parasternal outward movement due to a left atrium? Why?

    ANS: In severe chronic mitral regurgitation (MR). The left atrium is a mid-chest structure (i.e., it is not really a left atrium but a posterior atrium). (See figure on p. 100.)

3. How can you tell whether or not an expanding left atrium due to severe chronic MR is the cause of a marked left parasternal movement?

    ANS: Compare the LV apical movement with the left parasternal movement by placing a finger on each. A left atrial lift will begin and end slightly

later than the LV thrust. Right ventricular movement will begin and end
at the same time or even before the LV.

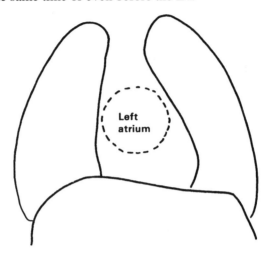

The "left" atrium is really a posterosuperior atrium, since it
is behind and above the right atrium. Although it is slightly to
the left of the right atrium, it is a midline structure.

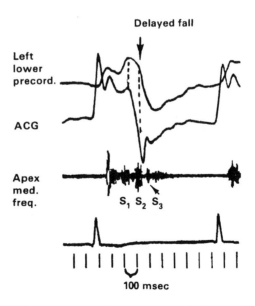

The left lower parasternal area movement shows a delayed
fall in comparison with the apical impulse in this patient with
severe chronic rheumatic MR.

X-RAY EVALUATION OF CARDIAC SIZE ───────────────

1. How is determination of cardiac size by X-ray usually calculated?

    ANS: By cardiothoracic (C/T) ratios. Fifty percent is considered by most radiologists to be the upper limit of normal.

2. How can we overcome the falsely normal C/T ratios in subjects who are short and underweight, or the falsely high C/T ratios in subjects who are overweight?

    ANS: By the use of the height and weight tables of Ungerleider and Clark [4].

3. How can you measure cardiac volume to derive a more accurate cardiac size than by any other X-ray method?

    ANS: The cardiac volume uses the lateral chest film and body surface area. The length dimension (L) is measured in centimeters from the junction of the superior vena cave and right atrium to the cardiac apex. The broad diameter (B) is measured from the junction of the right atrium and diaphragm to the junction of the pulmonary artery and left atrial appendage. The lateral dimension (D) is the greatest horizontal cardiac lateral diameter

$$\text{Cardiac volume} = \frac{L \times B \times D}{\text{BSA}} \times 0.42$$

where BSA = body surface area. The 0.42 is the correction factor for a 6-ft distance of the heart from the film [5].

    Instead of using the tables (see p. 102), one may use the formula

$$\frac{\text{Weight}}{\text{Height}} \times 25 = \begin{array}{l} + 70 \text{ for males} \\ + 62 \text{ for females} \end{array}$$

    The answer is in mm and 10% above the average may be normal or slightly enlarged. If kilos and mm are used, multiply the weight by 2.2 and divide the height by 2.5.

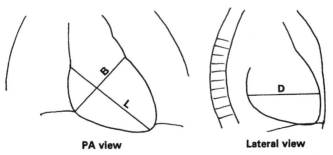

PA view   **Lateral view**

The upper normal values are 490 (cm³) for females and 540 (cm³) for males.

Theoretical transverse diameters of heart for various heights and weights

Table for determining percent deviation from average

Height

%Minus (−) %Plus (+)

(Light figures represent weights)

5'0"	1"	2"	3"	4"	5"	6"	7"	8"	9"	10"	11"	6'0"	1"	2"	3"	4"	5"	6"
83	85	86	87	89	90	92												
85	86	88	89	91	92	93	95											
87	88	90	91	92	94	95	97											
88	90	92	93	94	96	97	99	100										
90	92	93	95	96	98	99	101	102										
92	93	95	96	98	99	101	103	104	106									
94	95	98	100	101	103	104	106	108										
95	97	99	100	102	103	105	106	108	110	111								
97	99	100	102	104	105	107	108	110	112	113								
99	101	102	104	106	107	109	110	112	114	115	117							
101	102	104	106	108	109	111	113	114	116	118	119	121						
103	104	106	108	109	111	113	115	116	118	120	121	123	125					
105	106	108	110	111	113	115	117	118	120	122	124	125	127	129				
106	108	110	112	113	115	117	119	121	123	124	126	128	129	131	133			
108	110	112	114	115	117	119	121	123	125	126	128	130	132	133	135	137		
110	112	114	116	117	119	121	123	125	127	129	130	132	134	136	138	140	141	
112	114	116	118	120	121	123	125	127	129	131	133	134	136	138	140	142	144	146
114	116	118	120	122	124	125	127	129	131	133	135	137	139	141	143	145	147	149/151
116	118	120	122	124	126	128	129	131	133	135	137	139	141	143	145	147	149	151
118	120	122	124	126	128	130	132	134	136	138	140	142	143	145	147	149	151	153
120	122	124	126	128	130	132	134	136	138	140	142	144	146	148	150	152	154	156
122	124	126	128	130	132	134	136	138	140	142	144	146	148	150	152	154	156	159
124	126	128	130	132	134	136	138	140	143	145	147	149	151	153	155	157	159	161
126	128	130	132	134	136	139	141	143	145	147	149	151	153	155	157	160	162	164
128	130	132	134	137	139	141	143	145	147	149	152	154	156	158	160	162	164	166
130	132	134	137	139	141	143	145	147	150	152	154	156	158	160	163	165	167	169
132	134	137	139	141	143	145	148	150	152	154	156	159	161	163	165	167	170	172
134	137	139	141	143	146	148	150	152	154	157	159	161	163	166	168	170	172	175
136	139	141	143	146	148	150	152	155	157	159	161	164	166	168	171	173	175	177
139	141	143	146	148	150	152	155	157	159	162	164	166	169	171	173	176	178	180
141	143	145	148	150	152	155	157	160	162	164	167	169	171	174	176	178	181	183
143	145	148	150	152	155	157	160	162	164	167	169	172	174	176	179	181	183	186
145	148	150	152	155	157	160	162	164	167	169	172	174	177	179	181	184	186	189
147	150	152	155	157	160	162	165	167	169	172	174	177	179	182	184	187	189	192
150	152	155	157	160	162	165	167	169	172	174	177	179	182	184	187	189	192	194
152	154	157	159	162	164	167	169	172	175	177	180	182	185	187	190	192	195	197
154	157	159	162	164	167	169	172	175	177	180	182	185	187	190	193	195	198	200
156	159	162	164	167	169	172	175	177	180	182	185	188	190	193	195	198	201	203
159	161	164	167	169	172	174	177	180	182	185	188	190	193	196	198	201	204	206
161	164	166	169	172	174	177	180	182	185	188	190	193	196	198	201	204	206	209
163	166	169	171	174	177	180	182	185	188	190	193	196	199	201	204	207	209	212
166	168	171	174	177	179	182	185	188	190	193	196	199	201	204	207	210	212	215
168	171	174	176	179	182	185	188	190	193	196	199	202	204	207	210	213	216	218
170	173	176	179	182	184	187	190	193	196	199	202	204	207	210	213	216	219	221
173	176	178	181	184	187	190	193	196	199	201	204	207	210	213	216	219	222	224
175	178	181	184	187	190	193	196	198	201	204	207	210	213	216	219	222	225	228
178	180	183	186	189	192	195	198	201	204	207	210	213	216	219	222	225	228	231
180	183	186	189	192	195	198	201	204	207	210	213	216	219	222	225	228	231	234
182	185	188	192	195	198	201	204	207	210	213	216	219	222	225	228	231	234	237
185	188	191	194	197	200	203	206	210	213	216	219	222	225	228	231	234	237	240
187	191	194	197	200	203	206	209	212	215	219	222	225	228	231	234	237	240	243
190	193	196	199	203	206	209	212	215	218	222	225	228	231	234	237	241	244	247
192	196	199	202	205	208	212	215	218	221	224	228	231	234	237	241	244	247	250
195	198	201	205	208	211	214	218	221	224	227	231	234	237	240	244	247	250	253
198	201	204	207	211	214	217	221	224	227	230	234	237	240	244	247	250	253	257
200/206	203/210	207/213	210/216	213/220	217/223	220/227	224/230	227/233	230/236	233/240	237/243	240/247	243/250	247/254	250/257	253/260	257/264	260
216	219	222	226	229	233	236	239	243	246	249	253	256	260	263	267	270		
225	229	232	236	239	243	246	249	253	256	260	263	267	270					
235	239	242	246	249	253	256	260	263	267	270								
245	249	252	256	259	263	266	270	274	277									
255	259	263	266	270	273	277	281											
259	262	266	270	273	277	280	284											
269	273	277	280	284	287													
273	276	280	284	287	291													

Table for determining percent deviation from average:

25	20	15	10	5	▼	5	10	15	20	25
75	80	85	90	95	100	105	110	115	120	125
76	81	86	91	96	101	106	111	116	121	126
77	82	87	92	97	102	107	112	117	122	128
77	82	88	93	98	103	108	113	118	124	129
78	83	88	94	99	104	109	114	120	125	130
79	84	89	95	100	105	110	116	121	126	131
80	85	90	95	101	106	111	117	122	127	133
80	86	91	96	102	107	112	118	123	128	134
81	86	92	97	103	108	113	119	124	130	135
82	87	93	98	104	109	114	120	125	131	136
83	88	94	99	105	110	116	121	127	132	138
83	89	94	100	105	111	117	122	128	133	139
84	90	95	101	106	112	118	123	129	134	140
85	90	96	102	107	113	119	124	130	136	141
86	91	97	103	108	114	120	125	131	137	143
86	92	98	104	109	115	121	127	132	138	144
87	93	99	104	110	116	122	128	133	139	145
88	94	99	105	111	117	123	129	135	140	146
89	94	100	106	112	118	124	130	136	142	148
89	95	101	107	113	119	125	131	137	143	149
90	96	102	108	114	120	126	132	138	144	150
91	97	103	109	115	121	127	133	139	145	151
92	98	104	110	116	122	128	134	140	146	153
92	98	105	111	117	123	129	135	141	148	154
93	99	105	112	118	124	130	136	143	149	155
94	100	106	113	119	125	131	138	144	150	156
95	101	107	114	120	126	132	139	145	151	158
95	102	108	114	121	127	133	140	146	152	159
96	102	109	115	122	128	134	141	147	154	160
97	103	110	116	123	129	135	142	148	155	161
98	104	111	117	124	130	137	143	150	156	163
98	105	111	118	124	131	138	144	151	157	164
99	106	112	119	125	132	139	145	152	158	165
100	106	113	120	126	133	140	146	153	160	166
101	107	114	121	127	134	141	147	154	161	168
101	108	115	122	128	135	142	149	155	162	169
102	109	116	122	129	136	143	150	156	163	170
103	110	116	123	130	136	144	151	158	164	171
104	110	117	124	131	138	144	152	159	166	173
104	111	118	125	132	139	146	153	160	167	174
105	112	119	126	133	140	147	154	161	168	175
106	113	120	127	134	141	148	155	162	169	176
107	114	121	128	135	142	149	156	163	170	178
107	114	122	129	136	143	150	157	164	172	179
108	115	122	130	137	144	151	158	166	173	180
109	116	123	131	138	145	152	160	167	174	181
110	117	124	131	139	146	153	161	168	175	183
110	118	125	132	140	147	154	162	169	176	184
111	118	126	133	141	148	155	163	170	177	185
112	119	127	134	142	149	156	164	171	179	186
113	120	128	135	143	150	158	165	173	180	188
113	121	128	136	143	151	159	166	174	181	189
114	122	129	137	144	152	160	167	175	182	190
115	122	130	138	145	153	161	168	176	184	191
116	123	131	139	146	154	162	169	177	185	193
116	124	132	140	147	155	163	171	178	186	194
117	125	133	140	148	156	164	172	179	187	195
118	126	133	141	149	157	165	173	181	188	196
118	126	134	142	150	158	166	174	182	190	198
119	127	135	143	151	159	167	175	183	191	199
120	128	136	144	152	160	168	176	184	192	200
121	129	137	145	153	161	169	177	185	193	201
122	130	138	146	154	162	170	178	186	194	203
122	130	138	146	154	162	170	178	187	196	204
123	131	139	148	156	164	172	180	189	197	205

Actual Predicted Diameter (mm) Actual

The heart is usually enlarged if the width is 10% greater than the average prediction, which is shown in the boldface vertical column on the right. Subtract 8 mm for women, since this table was derived from thousands of male insurance applicants. (*Personal communication from Dr. H. E. Ungerleider.*)

DIAGNOSIS OF VENTRICULAR HYPERTROPHY
BY PHYSICAL EXAMINATION OF THE PRECORDIUM _____

Terminology Problems

1. What are the differences between cardiac hypertrophy, dilatation, enlargement, and overload?

ANS: The term *hypertrophy* refers to the thickening of the ventricular chambers. *Dilatation* refers to an increase in chamber volume. The terms *enlargement* and *overload* are not specific because they refer to either hypertrophy and/or dilatation. However, enlargement tends to be used as a synonym for dilatation.

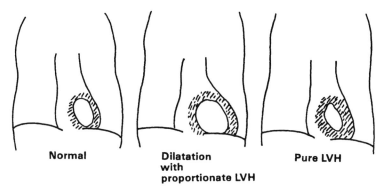

| Normal | Dilatation with proportionate LVH | Pure LVH |

Pure LVH causes an encroachment inward on the cavity and has been called "concentric" hypertrophy. Dilatation with proportionate hypertrophy has been called "eccentric" hypertrophy but is a confusing term that is best avoided.

2. What is meant by concentric vs eccentric hypertrophy?

ANS: *Concentric hypertrophy* refers to uniform hypertrophy of the ventricle. The opposite of concentric used to be *eccentric hypertrophy*, which, unfortunately, has many meanings. Eccentric hypertrophy has been applied to hearts with asymmetric septal hypertrophy, to dilated hearts that shifted the center eccentrically to the left, and to dilated hearts in which the hypertrophy was not proportional to the degree of dilatation. It should be apparent that the term eccentric hypertrophy should be avoided.

Note: Proportionate hypertrophy accompanies almost all chronically dilated ventricles.

The LV Impulse in Left Ventricular Hypertrophy (LVH)

1. How can you establish by palpation that an LV apex beat is normal, i.e., that there is no hypertrophy, dilatation, or loss of compliance?

   ANS: In the supine and left lateral decubitus positions the normal apex beat rises in systole and falls away rapidly to reach the S_2 at the bottom of the fall or even before the last one-third of systole. This is not a visual phenomenon, so only compare what you hear with what you *feel*.

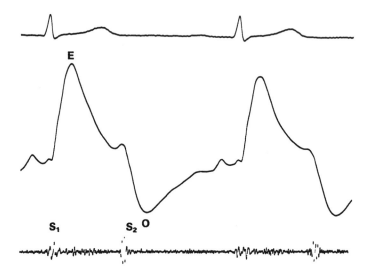

This depicts a normal apex impulse (apex cardiogram, or ACG) recorded over the apex beat with the subject in the left lateral decubitus position. The fingers feel the E–O slope as a purely systolic retraction. The S_2–O portion of the slope is so short and rapid that the O nadir is perceived as ending at the S_2. The end-systolic hump of the ACG is not perceived by palpation as interrupting the E–O slope.

2. What characteristics are imparted to an apex beat by a hypertrophied LV?

   ANS: a. It will be sustained.
         b. It may have a presystolic A wave or atrial hump.
         c. It may have a midsystolic dip.

3. What is meant by a sustained apex beat?

   ANS: It is one that remains outward throughout systole and begins to go away only with the second heart sound. This is usually detected with the patient in the left lateral decubitus position.

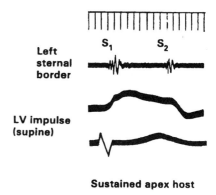

If you imagine a sound shortly after the S_2, the sustained apex beat will seem fall onto it rather than onto the S_2.

Note: The term *heave* is often used to describe a large area and amplitude of sustained movement.

4. What is the most common mimic of the sustained apical impulse of LV dilatation?

   ANS: A ventricular aneurysm involving the apex.

   Note: a. In the absence of LVH or an aneurysm, a sustained apex beat suggests a depressed ejection fraction.
   b. Complete absence of the pericardium can also not only produce a sustained apical impulse but can displace it into the axilla.

5. How can the degree of aortic regurgitation (AR) be judged by the degree of sustaining?

   ANS: With mild to moderate AR, the impulse may be overactive but will fall to its lowest level before the S_2. When the AR is moderately severe or severe, proportionate hypertrophy will cause the apex beat to be sustained.

The A Wave or Palpable Atrial Hump

1. How does a cineangiogram show the effect of a contracting atrium on the ventricle?

   ANS: With contrast material in the LV, a cineangiogram can show that the LV suddenly expands at the end of diastole in response to atrial contraction.

2. When is this end-diastolic or presystolic expansion of the LV palpable?

   ANS: The normal A wave is not palpable. Only a very strong left atrial contraction can expand the LV with enough force to cause a palpable presystolic hump on the LV impulse.

Note: If the atrial hump, or A wave, is too close to the outward movement of
the ventricular contraction, it may be impalpable even if it is very high.
This can be caused by a short P–R interval.

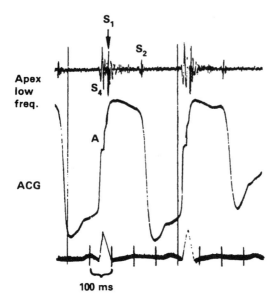

A short P–R of about 80 ms due
to a preexcitation abnormality has
caused the atrial hump (A) to be
too close to the major ventricular
movement to be palpable.

3. What is the cause of a left atrial contraction strong enough to make a palpable
LV hump at the LV impulse?

   ANS: Severe loss of LV **compliance** (i.e., loss of distensibility of the LV).

   Note: The strong atrial contraction effect on the LV is often called the "atrial
   kick" or booster-pump effect. The reason for this is that the expansion
   of the LV just before its contraction produces an increased energy of
   ventricular contraction via the **Starling effect**. The A wave has the same
   significance as does the S_4.

4. How does the left atrium "get the message" to contract harder when the LV is
stiffer?

   ANS: In diastole, the mitral valve is open and the left atrium and ventricle are
   in continuity (i.e., they are, in effect, an atrioventricle). When the ventricle is stiff, the atrioventricle is also stiff, and when blood pours into a
   stiff chamber, the pressure rises steeply. If the atrium is under high pressure at the end of diastole, then, due to the Starling effect, it will contract more strongly.

   Note: The atrium will hypertrophy in response to its continued strong con-
   tractions and will then contribute to the stiffness of the atrioventricle.

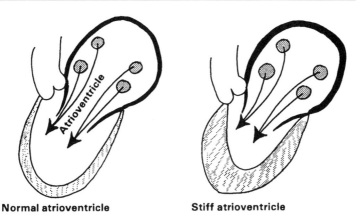

Normal atrioventricle   **Stiff atrioventricle**

A stiff ventricle must be transmitting its loss of compliance to the atrium during diastole when the AV valves open.

5. What is the most common cause of chronic increased stiffness of the LV? What is the next most common?

ANS: LVH, secondary to hypertension. The next most common cause is coronary disease (i.e., the confluent patchy areas of fibrosis or infarction plus the tendency to hypertrophy of the remaining healthy myocardium can cause a stiff LV).

6. Why is it important to palpate for an A wave?

ANS: The S_4 may be inaudible, or the S_4, S_1 may be mistaken for an S_1, ejection sound. You may be able to palpate an A wave but not hear an S_4 because the frequency of vibrations may be too low for audibility but not for palpation.

7. What does an atrial kick feel like to the palpating fingers?

ANS: When it is strong and far from the ventricle outward movement, it feels like a double outward movement. When it is slight or close to the ventricular outward movement, it feels like a notch, vibration, or hesitation on the apical upstroke.

Note: These movements are best felt by the part of the hand near the fingertips with the patient in the left lateral decubitus position. Occasionally a suspected faint atrial kick can be confirmed by observing a double outward movement of the patient's skin, or of your stethoscope on the LV impulse. An atrial hump may only be felt with light finger pressure unless there is much muscle or fat, in which case it will be necessary to press firmly.

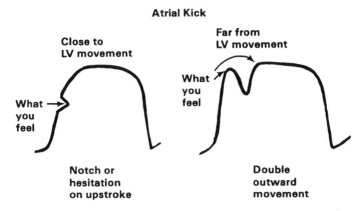

If only a notch or slight hesitation is present on the upstroke, the tips of the fingers must be used to perceive it. If a large double movement is felt, it must be distinguished from a mid-systolic dip.

The Midsystolic Dip

1. With which abnormality do you often find a mid-systolic dip in the presence of LVH?

   ANS: Hypertrophic obstructive cardiomyopathy (HOCM).

2. What kind of impulse may be imparted to the apex beat of a patient with severe HOCM if an A wave is also present?

   ANS: A triple outward movement (known by some as a "triple ripple"). This is almost pathognomonic of HOCM).

3. Which valvular abnormality may have a mid-systolic dip without LVH?

   ANS: A prolapsed mitral valve. An S₄ or a click and murmur quickly differentiates the cause of the dip.

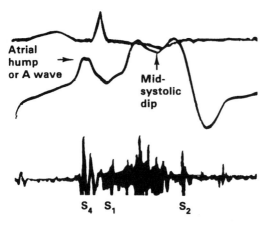

This apex impulse tracing (apex cardiogram) is from a 45-year-old man with HOCM. The atrial hump and the midsystolic dip give an impression of a triple outward movement.

Right Ventricular Hypertrophy (RVH)

1. What are the characteristics of a normal left parasternal impulse?

    ANS: It consists of a tiny inward (posterior) movement throughout most of systole due to the emptying of the RV. In children and in some adults, there is a smaller-amplitude initial outward movement of short duration, probably due to a change in shape of the RV during isovolumic contraction.

2. How does the left parasternal impulse caused by the RVH or pulmonary stenosis (PS) or pulmonary hypertension differ from normal?

    ANS: It is a systolic outward movement with its peak in early or mid-systole.

    Note: a. The site of maximum RV impulse in patients with PS is often a few centimeters away from the parasternal area and may even be in the mid-left thorax.

    b. In valvular PS the parasternal impulse may be as high as the third left interspace, whereas in infundibular stenosis the impulse is confined to the fourth or fifth interspace.

    c. A descending aortic aneurysm can also cause an anterior systolic movement of the sternum and parasternal areas.

3. What is the significance of feeling the impulse of a dilated pulmonary artery in the second left interspace in a patient with RVH?

    ANS: A palpable pulmonary artery movement is usually secondary to a dilated RV, as in ASD or primary pulmonary hypertension. The dilated pulmonary artery is best palpated in full held expiration, with the patient either supine or at various degrees of chest elevation. It is often better seen than palpated, and gentle pressure should be applied first. In patients with narrow anteroposterior diameters, a normal pulmonary trunk can sometimes be both visible and palpable.

REFERENCES

1. Sleight, P. Unilateral elevation of the internal jugular pulse. *Br. Heart J.* 24:726, 1962.
2. Fukuda, N., et al. Phono-mechano- and echocardiographic studies of patients with funnel chest, especially on the changes of the jugular phlebogram and interventricular septal motion. *J. Cardiogr.* 11:161,1981.
3. Dressler, W. Clinical aids to cardiac diagnosis. Grune and Stratton, New York, NY, 1970.
4. Ungerleider, H. E., Clark, C. P. A. A study of the transverse diameter of the heart with prediction tables. *Am. J. Heart* 17:92, 1939.
5. Keats, T. E., and Enge, I. P. Cardiac mensuration by cardiac volume method. *Radiology* 85:850, 1965.

6 The Stethoscope

THE BELL CHEST PIECE

1. What is the relation between the tautness (stiffness) of a membrane that collects sound from the chest wall and the ability of the membrane to transmit high or low frequencies?

    ANS: The tauter the membrane, the higher is its natural frequency of oscillation and the more efficient it is at higher frequencies.

    Note: The terms *frequency* and *pitch* are usually used interchangeably. However, frequency refers to the number of oscillations per second made by a sound-producing structure, while pitch is what you hear when those vibrations act on your hearing apparatus.

2. What is the ideal membrane to apply to a chest wall in order to bring out low frequencies?

    ANS: A membrane that is as loose and flabby as possible.

3. How does the use of a bell chest piece fit into these acoustical laws?

    ANS: The bell allows you to use the skin as a flabby diaphragm. The skin can be turned into a taut diaphragm if enough pressure is applied to the skin to produce pain.

4. Which chest piece diameter picks up the most sound, a very small one or a very large one?

    ANS: A very large one. The ability of a chest piece to collect sound is proportional to its diameter.

5. Which chest piece diameter picks up low frequencies better, a small one or a large one?

    ANS: A large one.

6. How much pressure should be applied with a bell chest piece?

    ANS: Just enough to prevent room-noise leak. Any more pressure will tighten the skin and tend to damp out the low frequencies.

    Note: An exception to this occurs when you are listening for an S_4. Firm pressure with the bell will sometimes bring out an S_4.

7. What is the relationship between the internal volume of a stethoscope (air space enclosed by the chest piece and tubing) and the loudness of the transmitted sound?

    ANS: There is an inverse relationship—i.e., the smaller the internal volume, the greater is the loudness of the sound.

8. What bell design will give the smallest internal volume and the largest diameter?

    ANS: A shallow shell rather than a deep cone.

    Note: It is believed by some cardiologists, with no explanation or testing other than their own ears, that a third chest piece consisting of a large-diameter corrugated diaphragm applied with light pressure (actually only the weight of the three-headed stethoscope) is sometimes best for hearing low frequencies. They still advise having a bell handy, however, both because a small bell is needed for auscultation in small places, such as the supraclavicular fossa or between the ribs on a bony chest, and because the large bell is occasionally superior for certain low frequencies.

9. What kind of murmurs and sounds are best heard with the bell?

    ANS: Murmurs: diastolic murmurs through atrioventricular valves (mitral and tricuspid). Sounds: the diastolic sounds known as the S_3 and S_4.

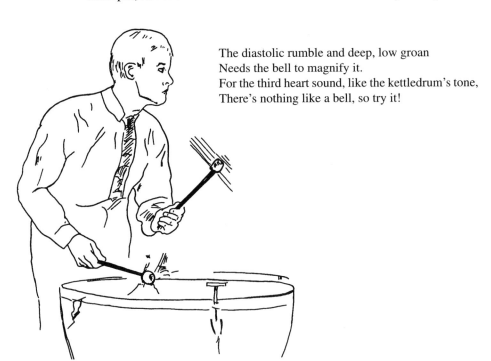

The diastolic rumble and deep, low groan
Needs the bell to magnify it.
For the third heart sound, like the kettledrum's tone,
There's nothing like a bell, so try it!

Note: The kettledrum (tympany) is bell-shaped and is also used to bring out the low-frequency, booming tones.

Adults can hear frequencies of up to 14,000 cycles per second (cps). However, since cardiac sound does not extend much above 1,000 cps, loss of ability to hear frequencies above 3,000 cps, which is the usual type of hearing loss in older physicians, should not interfere with the hearing of any cardiac sounds or murmurs.

THE SMOOTH DIAPHRAGM

1. What is meant by "masking" of sounds?

    ANS: Masking of sounds refers to the inability to hear a sound well because of interference by another loud sound occurring just before it or just after it.

2. Do low frequencies mask high ones easily?

    ANS: Yes, unless the lower frequencies are very widely separated in pitch from the higher frequencies or are relatively soft.

3. What is the purpose of the smooth, stiff diaphragm?

    ANS: To damp out low frequencies and unmask high frequencies. If the resonance frequency of the diaphragm happens to be the same as that of the murmur, it may actually amplify the murmur.

    Note: a. Amplification of sound may also be due to the summation of reflected or standing waves in the tubing. Different tubing lengths therefore may amplify different frequencies.
    b. Although a bell will bring out low frequencies considerably better than a diaphragm, high-frequency sounds and murmurs are actually heard almost as well with the bell as with the diaphragm.

4. Why not use the bell chest piece as a diaphragm by merely applying pressure, thus eliminating the need for two chest pieces?

    ANS: The stretched skin is an inefficient diaphragm for filtering out low frequencies. The skin does not become still enough to be a good filter.

    Note: a. Do not use X-ray film as a substitute for a damaged diaphragm. X-ray film has been shown to be about as good as no diaphragm at all for filtering out low frequencies. It is not stiff enough.
    b. A greater degree of pressure variation with the diaphragm has been attained through prestressing a nylon diaphragm by bowing it slightly forward. A small raised area in the center of the diaphragm can further increase the tension by exerting pressure against the skin [1].

5. Which murmurs and sounds are usually heard well only with the stiff, smooth diaphragm?

     ANS: Murmurs: the soft aortic and pulmonary diastolic murmur and the soft mitral regurgitation murmur. Sounds: splitting of first or second heart sounds and nonejection clicks.

6. Why is it very difficult to hear the splitting of heart sounds with a bell?

     ANS: There are so many low-frequency "reverberations" surrounding each component that the ear cannot separate them if the splitting is close. The ear can separate two short, high-frequency sounds placed close to each other more easily than it can separate two prolonged low- or medium-frequency sounds.

THE TUBING

1. Which frequencies are attenuated (damped) by too long a tubing?

     ANS: High frequencies. The low frequencies are relatively unaffected by tube length.

2. What is the shortest compromise length that will bring out high frequencies and still not be too short for comfort?

     ANS: A length of 12 in. (30 cm). However, 15 in. (37.5 cm) is a good compromise between the ideal 12 in. and the usual 20–22 in. that are commercially available.

3. How can the thickness of the tubing affect auscultation?

     ANS: The thicker the tube, the better is the elimination of room noise. A vinyl tube has been found to be better than rubber for this purpose.

4. Which is more efficient, a single tube or a double tube?

     ANS: The single-tube stethoscopes appear at first glance to be more efficient because they eliminate the necessity for binding parallel tubes together to prevent collision sounds, and they are more flexible and portable. However, tests have shown that the double tube is more efficient for high frequencies, because it allows less interference from reflected waves [2]. However, a single tube attenuates only frequencies of over 400 cps, which suggests that only the very softest and highest-pitched murmurs will be missed by using a single tube.

AIR LEAKS AND EAR TIPS

1. How important are air leaks at either the earpiece changeover valve or chest piece?

    ANS: The greatest impairment of the efficiency of a stethoscope is the air leak. Room noise due to air leaks tends to mask high frequencies more than low ones.

2. How can you test for air leaks at the chest piece or changeover valve?

    ANS: a. Blow into one tube while occluding the opposite earpiece and tubing. Your fingers will feel the air escaping.

    b. If withdrawing the chest piece quickly from the precordium produces a change in pressure that is painful to the ear, an air leak, if present, is probably unimportant.

3. Why may small ear tips become partially obstructed when being inserted into the ear?

    ANS: The usual stethoscope headpieces are designed to point the ear tips slightly anteriorly. If the ear tips are too small, their aperture may impinge partially or completely against the cartilaginous meatus, which points backward.

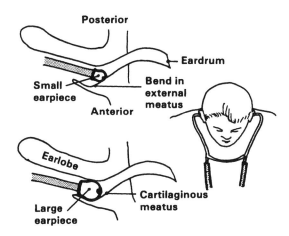

Headpieces are designed to point the ear tips slightly anteriorly. Small ear tips can therefore be partly occluded against the backward-directed meatus.

SUMMARY OF GOOD STETHOSCOPE CHARACTERISTICS _____

1. A shallow bell with a large diameter for low frequencies.
2. A smooth, stiff, thin diaphragm for high frequencies.
3. A pediatric-sized bell and diaphragm accessories.
4. An internally smooth vinyl tubing, not over 12 in. (30 cm) long and $^3/_{16}$ in. (4.6 mm) in internal diameter.
5. Double tubing with some method of binding the tubes together.
6. The largest ear tips possible.
7. Metal headpieces that can be rotated so that the ear tips can be pointed in the most comfortable direction.

REFERENCES _____

1. Howell, W. L., and Aldridge, C. F. The effect of stethoscope-applied pressure in auscultation. *Circulation* 32:430,1965.
2. Ertel, P Y., et al. Stethoscope acoustics 1. The doctor and his stethoscope. *Circulation* 34:889, 1966.

7 Diagramming and Grading Heart Sounds and Murmurs

THE AUSCULTOGRAM

A graphic method for illustrating auscultatory findings is offered here, not only as a means of keeping records as conveniently and efficiently as possible, but also as an aid in learning auscultation. One such "auscultogram" (see figures) can equal a 629-word description of the auscultatory findings. The graph can tell the story at a glance once the symbols are understood.

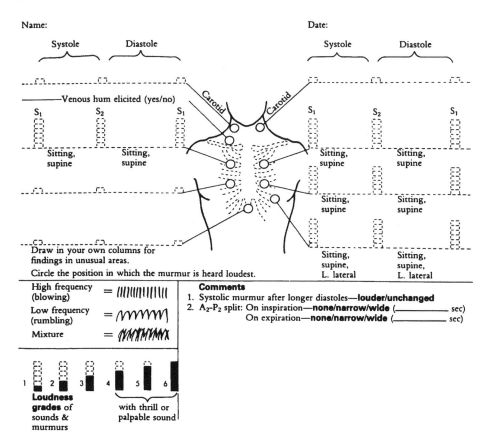

Filling in such auscultograms serves a self-teaching function in training a person in auscultation, because one is forced to dissect out and listen separately to each component of the cycle, a method that is the hallmark of a good auscultator. Although listening to the total effect of all the sounds and murmurs as a single unit is also important, beginners tend to listen this way to the exclusion of the dissection method.

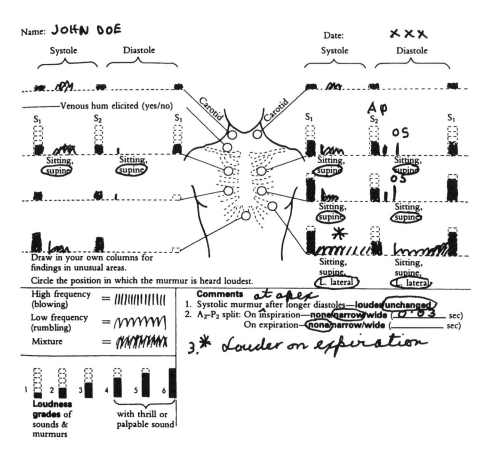

The writing and listening should be done simultaneously (i.e., with the stethoscope in one hand and a pen in the other, the auscultator fills in the auscultogram). The auscultogram is used for the purpose of improving the ability to auscultate and providing an accurate record; the art of fine auscultation should not be a memory test. Performing auscultation is one of the few times when it is best for a right-handed physician to carry out the examination from the patient's left side, because this position allows the stethoscope to be held with he left hand while writing with the right.

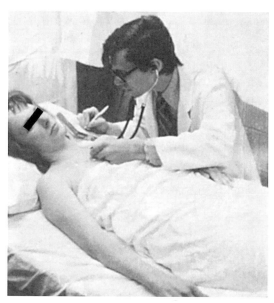

Simultaneous writing and listening is the key to this method
of ear training and accuracy of recording.

It is convenient to print auscultogram pads that are small enough to fit on about
half a hospital chart page. The auscultograms illustrated at the beginning of this
chapter are the actual size.

GRADING OF HEART SOUNDS AND MURMURS

Freeman and Levine in 1933 introduced the grading of murmurs up to 6 [1].
However, they did not describe either how to tell grade 3 from grade 4 or the psycho-
logical approach to grade 1 murmurs.

Grading 1 to 6 is now generally accepted according to the following criteria,
which serve for heart sounds as well as murmurs.

Grade 1   So soft that you must "tune in" to hear it. Tuning in means
            that you must know what to expect before you can hear it.
            Then you can eliminate room noise psychologically and
            try to hear something that you can already picture in your
            mind. A grade 1 murmur or heart sound has been defined as
            one that a medical student cannot hear. There is some truth
            in this, because a student often does not know what a soft
            blowing regurgitant murmur sounds like. You cannot
            "tune in" to nothing.

Grade 2	A soft murmur or sound that anyone can hear.
Grade 3	A loud murmur or sound that is not palpable.
Grade 4	A loud murmur or sound that is palpable. When you feel a murmur, you are said to be feeling a "**thrill**." When you feel a heart sound, you are said to be feeling a "tap," or simply a "palpable sound."
Grade 5	A loud murmur that can be felt with the edge of the stethoscope, preferably with the diaphragm chest piece.
Grade 6	A murmur loud enough to be heard with the stethoscope slightly off the chest.

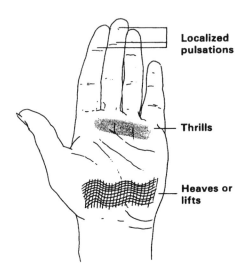

Localized pulsations

Thrills

Heaves or lifts

Although small localized movements are best perceived by the distal finger pads, thrills are best felt with the distal palm.

Note: **Thrills** and heart sounds are best perceived with the distal palm. One hand may be more sensitive than the other, so test each hand on any patient with a faint thrill or palpable sound to find your better hand.

REFERENCES

1. Levine, S. A., and Harvey, W. P. *Clinical Auscultation of the Heart.* Philadelphia: Saunders, 1959.

Boldface type indicates that the term is explained in the glossary.

8 The First Heart Sound (S₁)

PHYSIOLOGY OF THE FIRST SOUND COMPONENTS _____

1. Draw a left ventricular (LV) pressure curve.

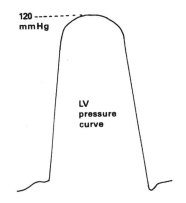

An LV pressure curve begins at a pressure of about 0 mmHg and rises to the same systolic pressure as in the aorta, i.e., normally about 120 mmHg.

2. Draw a left atrial pressure curve on the ventricular pressure curve and show where the mitral valve closes. Why does it close here?

ANS: The mitral valve closes when LV pressure rises above left atrial pressure, which is about 10 mmHg. If the left atrial pressure at the beginning of ventricular contraction is 10 mmHg, then as soon as the LV reaches a pressure of slightly more than 10 mmHg, the mitral valve will close.

The most important component of the S₁, which is the mitral component of M₁, occurs as the result of this valve closure, but the sound should not be thought of as due to the slapping together of leaflets. It is more probably due to sudden cessation of mitral valve flow at the time of maximum leaflet tension that occurs immediately after leaflet apposition, setting the entire cardiohemic system into vibration.

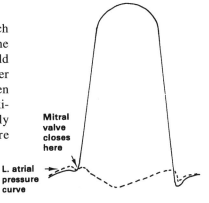

121

3. Draw an aortic pressure curve on the ventricular pressure curve and show where the aortic valve opens. (See question 4.)

4. When does the aortic valve open if the aortic diastolic pressure is 80 mmHg?

   ANS: The aortic valve opens when the LV pressure exceeds the aortic diastolic pressure of 80 mmHg.

   Note: The time between closure of the mitral valve and the opening of the aortic valve is the **isovolumic contraction** period.

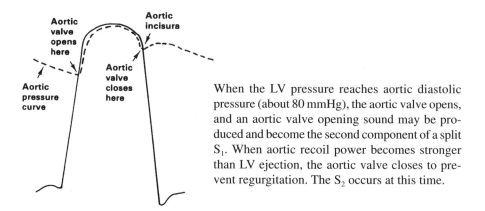

When the LV pressure reaches aortic diastolic pressure (about 80 mmHg), the aortic valve opens, and an aortic valve opening sound may be produced and become the second component of a split S_1. When aortic recoil power becomes stronger than LV ejection, the aortic valve closes to prevent regurgitation. The S_2 occurs at this time.

5. How do these pressure curves relate to the first heart sound, or S_1?

   ANS: The events associated with closure of the mitral valve and ejection of blood into the aorta are probably responsible for the two major components of the S_1. However, many cardiologists believe that the second major component of the split S_1 is due to closure of the tricuspid valve, ignoring the fact that mitral and tricuspid closure occur 0 02–0.03 s apart, which can be distinguished only with difficulty even by expert auscultators.

6. What are the components to the usual split of S_1?

   ANS: If the components are close together—fast enough to say "ta-da" as quickly as possible as if you were rolling the syllables on your tongue—they are probably due to mitral followed by tricuspid closure, i.e., M_1–T_1. If the components are fairly well separated, as in saying "pa-ta" as quickly as possible, then the components are probably mitral closure followed by aortic valve opening, or M_1–A_1 [1]. The second component of a wide split, or A_1, is more commonly known as an ejection sound, and it is occasionally so short and sharp that it is then known as an ejection click.

Boldface type indicates that the term is explained in the glossary.

7. When is it likely that tricuspid closure is the second component of a split S₁?

   ANS: a. Whenever the right ventricle (RV) has a volume or pressure over-
            load, as in ASD or in the presence of pulmonary hypertension.
         b. **Ebstein's anomaly**.

8. In what percentage of normal subjects is splitting of the S₁ audible?

   ANS: In about 85%.

THE M₁ PLUS AORTIC EJECTION SOUND AS THE CAUSE OF A SPLIT S₁

1. How long after the M₁ does the aortic ejection sound (A₁) occur in normal
   subjects?

   ANS: The usual A₁ occurs at the end of isovolumic contraction (i.e., about
        40–60 ms [0.04–0.06 s] after the M₁). To help you judge this normal
        split of the first sound interval, a 40-ms split takes as long as it does to
        say "pa-da" moderately quickly. The 60-ms split can be imitated by
        saying "pa-ta" as quickly as possible. (A 40- to 60-ms split is a moder-
        ately wide split.)

2. Which valvular abnormalities are the usual causes of an aortic ejection sound
   (or click)?

   ANS: a. A bicuspid aortic valve without stenosis. (Bicuspid valves may or
            may not become stenotic.)
         b. A stiff aortic valve, such as that occurring in AS or hypertension.

   Note: Hypertension may stretch the aortic root, causing the cusps to become
           taut and therefore to open with a sharp sound.

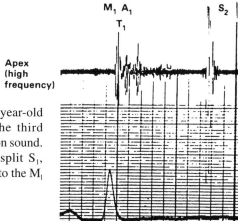

This phonocardiogram is from a 40-year-old woman with mild hypertension. The third component is probably an aortic ejection sound. This sounded simply like a widely split S₁, probably because the T₁ was too close to the M₁ to be audible.

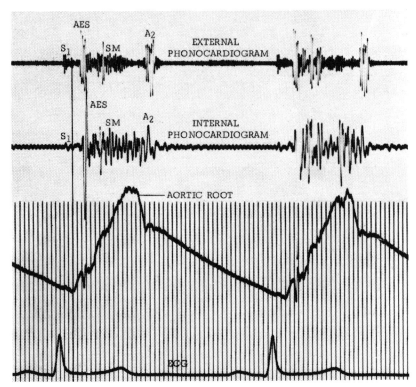

Aortic root tracing from a 23-year-old man with congenital AS taken with a catheter-tip electromanometer so that there are no tubing delays. The aortic ejection sound (AES) is coincident with the moment of peak opening of the valve. SM = systolic murmur.

3. What features suggest that the aortic ejection sound or click, as in **aortic stenosis,** is due to an opening snap of the aortic valve and not merely to forceful ejection into the aorta?

   ANS: a. It disappears with severe calcification of the aortic valve; conversely, the louder the sound the more mobile the valve can be shown to be.

   b. It is not a feature of supravalvular AS or of obstruction below the valve, i.e., hypertrophic obstructive cardiomyopathy (HOCM) or discrete subvalvular stenosis.

4. Where is the aortic ejection sound best heard?

   ANS: The ejection sound is well heard wherever aortic events are best heard, i.e., anywhere in a straight line or "sash area" from the second right interspace to the apex. The ejection click of AS, however, is most often heard best at the apex because the AS murmur may be loud enough elsewhere to obscure the click.

5. What additional information does an aortic ejection sound give you in the presence of AS?

    ANS: a. It helps to locate the site of the AS because only valvular AS characteristically has an audible ejection sound.

    b. The absence of an ejection sound in valvular AS implies a calcified aortic valve. A calcified valve of that degree is highly correlated with a gradient of more than 50 mmHg.

6. What features may suggest that an aortic ejection sound is due to a bicuspid aortic valve (nonstenotic)?

    ANS: a. If it is loud, especially if it is louder than the M_1, and is associated with a louder A_2 than normal.

    b. If it is associated with aortic regurgitation (AR), usually of only mild to moderate degree. (AR is commonly associated with a bicuspid aortic valve.)

    Note: A bicuspid aortic valve may calcify in patients over 50 years old and lead to AS of any degree, or it may remain nonstenotic permanently.

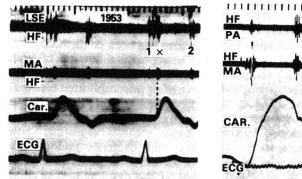 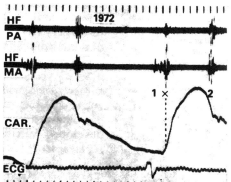

This patient with a bicuspid aortic valve showed (on the left) a triple S_1 of M_1 T_1 A_1 in 1953, at age 28. Twenty-five years later the late aortic ejection pound (labeled X) is louder than the M_1, and no stenosis has developed.

THE PULMONARY EJECTION SOUND

Ejection Sound in Pulmonary Stenosis (PS)

1. What proof can be offered that the ejection sound heard in valvular PS it an opening sound of the pulmonary valve?

    ANS: a. It is not present in pure infundibular stenosis.

    b. It occurs at the peak of opening of the pulmonary valve on echocardiography.

2. Why does the pulmonary ejection sound tend to disappear with inspiration in valvular PS?

   ANS: The sudden upward movement of a dome-shaped pulmonary valve produces the sound. If the valve is already in the domed or near-domed position when the RV contracts, there will be no sound or only a soft sound. On inspiration, the increased blood drawn into the right atrium causes it to contract more strongly at the end of diastole. This raises the end-diastolic pressure in the RV just before the ventricle contracts to a level that may be higher than the pulmonary artery pressure. This is easy to understand if you realize that pulmonary artery diastolic pressure in PS may not be much more than 7 mmHg, and RV end-diastolic pressure in PS can easily exceed 7 mmHg. Thus the pulmonary valve will be raised into the domed position at the end of diastole if the end-diastolic pressure in the RV rises to 8 mmHg with a strong right atrial contraction.

   On expiration, the end-diastolic pressure in the RV falls, and the pulmonary valve is now in the down position at the beginning of RV systole. Ventricular contraction can now balloon the pulmonary valve upward into a dome, causing a click.

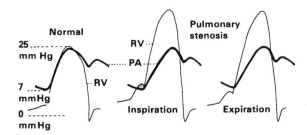

These RV and pulmonary artery pressure tracings show how inspiration can raise the end-diastolic RV pressure above pulmonary artery (PA) pressure because of a strong right atrial contraction plus a thick RV.

3. Why does the aortic ejection sound not change significantly with respiration?

   ANS: The end-diastolic pressure in the LV in AS, even when very high (the normal end-diastolic pressure is not much higher than 10 mmHg), can never exceed the usual diastolic pressure in the aorta (which is rarely ever lower than 50 mmHg). Therefore, expiration alone can never force the aortic valve into an upward domed position at the end of diastole.

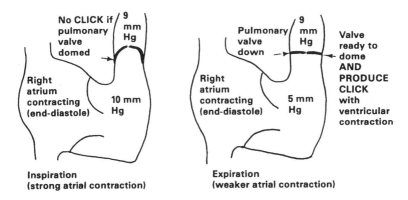

On the left is shown how right atrial contraction is assisted by inspiration in raising RV pressure higher than pulmonary artery pressure. This causes the pulmonary valve to dome upward before the RV contracts. On the right is depicted the effect of a reduction in RV diastolic pressure caused by expiration resulting in a downward position of the pulmonary valve when the RV begins to contract.

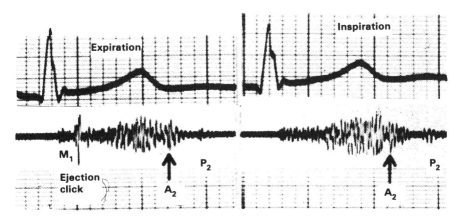

A high-frequency phonocardiogram from the third left interspace of a patient with PS and an RV pressure of 100 mmHg. The ejection sound tells you that the obstruction is valvular. Note that it disappears on inspiration.

Note: A pulmonic ejection sound tends to occur more often in mild to moderate stenosis, i.e., with RV pressures of not over 70 mmHg. (Normal RV systolic pressure is about 25 mmHg.)

4. Where is the pulmonary ejection sound best heard?

ANS: Wherever pulmonary sounds and murmurs are best heard, i.e., anywhere along the left sternal border.

Ejection Sound in Pulmonary Hypertension

1. Why is an ejection sound heard in pulmonary hypertension?

    ANS: The high pressure in the pulmonary artery may dilate the pulmonary artery root, and the valve ring will be stretched. The tautened cusps, opening at a very rapid rate, probably produce the sound or click.

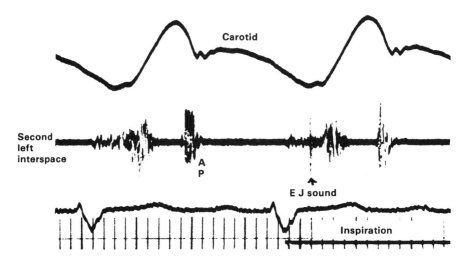

This high-frequency phonocardiogram and simultaneous carotid tracing is from a patient with severe pulmonary hypertension secondary to a VSD (**Eisenmenger syndrome**). Note that the pulmonary ejection (E J) sound does not diminish with inspiration.

2. How does an ejection sound heard in pulmonary hypertension differ from one heard in PS?

    ANS: In pulmonary hypertension the ejection sound is

      a. Often heard better lower down on the chest.
      b. Rarely changed by respiration.

Ejection Sounds in Idiopathic Dilatation of the Pulmonary Artery

1. How can you explain the ejection sound in idiopathic dilatation of the pulmonary artery if high pressure in the artery is not present to tighten the valve ring, and the pulmonary valve is not stenosed and therefore unable to produce an opening snap?

    ANS: Idiopathic dilatation of the pulmonary artery implies an abnormal artery with marked loss of elasticity. A jerky expansion of this lax pulmonary artery may cause a sudden sound or click.

LOUDNESS OF THE M$_1$

1. What controls the loudness of the M$_1$, besides chest wall shape and thickness or insulating effusion?

    ANS: a. The rate of rise of ventricular pressure at the time that it closes the mitral valve. The faster the rise at the time that the LV pressure exceeds left atrial pressure, the louder the M$_1$.

    b. The duration of LV contraction before it exceeds left atrial pressure. This is because the LV accelerates in the early phase of its contraction, and the longer the LV must contract before it can close the mitral valve, the louder the M$_1$.

    c. The stiffness of the mitral valve bellies. An immobile valve can produce little sound.

Ventricular Pressure Rise and M$_1$ Loudness

1. What is the physiologist's way of expressing the rate of rise of pressure?

    ANS: Delta *P*/delta *t* = change of pressure/change of time. This is usually shortened to *dP/dt*.

2. What is the relationship between the *dP/dt* of the LV and M$_1$ loudness?

    ANS: The greater the dP/dt (i.e., the faster the rate of LV pressure rise), the louder the M$_1$.

3. What can cause an increased *dP/dt* of the LV and therefore make the M$_1$ louder?

    ANS: Increased contractility due to positive inotropic agents such as catecholamines, sympathetic stimulation, digitalis, or thyroxine. Sympathetic stimulation is probably the cause of the loud M$_1$ in sinus tachycardia and in exercise.

4. What can decrease the *dP/dt* of the LV and therefore make the M$_1$ softer?

    ANS: Drugs such as beta blockers that decrease contractility.

    Note: a. These soft first sounds are often described as muffled because they have lost most of their high frequencies.

    b. Advancing age because of the decreasing *dP/dT*, their longer P–R and the increase in antero-posterior chest diameter.

The P–R Interval and M$_1$ Loudness

1. Why does a short P–R interval cause a loud M$_1$?

    ANS: The P controls the timing of atrial contraction, which raises left atrial (LA) pressure. The force of the contraction opens the mitral valve further at the end of diastole. The R controls the timing of ventricular contraction. If the P–R interval is short, ventricular contraction occurs so quickly after the atrium has contracted that the LA has not had time to relax (short X descent). Therefore, atrial pressure is still at a high level when the pressure in the LV exceeds it enough to close the mitral valve [2]. This means that the ventricle has a long time to contract before it overcomes the relatively high LA pressure. Therefore, the LV has time to accelerate to a rapid *dP/dt* part of its pressure curve by the time it closes the mitral valve. (See the accompanying figure.)

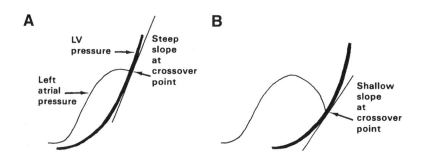

A. If the P–R interval is short, the LV contracts before the left atrium has had a chance to relax and drop its pressure. Therefore, the LV pressure will not exceed left atrial pressure until it has contracted for a long enough time to accelerate to a stage of rapid pressure rise by the time the mitral leaflets are closed. This produces an abrupt deceleration of forward flow and a loud sound.

B. If the P–R interval is long, the LV contracts later than at A, so that the left atrium has had time to drop to a low pressure when the LV pressure exceeds it. The pressure crossover point is on the slow part of the LV acceleration curve, and the valves are closed at a relatively slow rate, producing a soft sound.

2. Why does a long P–R interval cause a soft M_1?

   ANS: The delayed LV contraction gives the LA pressure a chance to drop to low levels (deep X descent) by the time the LV begins to contract. Thus LV pressure will exceed LA pressure at the very early slow part of its acceleration curve [2].

   Note: a. It has usually been taught that the reason for the loud M_1 with a short P–R is that the mitral leaflets are wide open at the time of the LV contraction onset—i.e., atrial relaxation, which is known to be able to close mitral valves by a kind of suction effect [3], has not had much time to act. The analogy of a wide-open door making more noise when it closes than does a slightly open door is often used but is not valid unless the door is made to accelerate as it closes.

b. The paradox of a long P–R interval and a loud S₁ is seen in mitral stenosis (MS) and also in **Ebstein's anomaly**. In the latter, the M₁ may actually be very soft, but the second component of the S₁ may be loud, short, and clicking because it is caused by a closure of a large deformed anterior leaflet of the tricuspid valve. Because this leaflet has been likened to a large sail flapping in the breeze, this loud T₁ has been called a sail sound. This sound often increases with inspiration and is usually associated with a very late tricuspid opening snap.

c. In sudden severe aortic regurgitation the mitral valve may be closed in mid-diastole and is associated with a soft or inaudible S₁.

d. A soft S₁ in the presence of an S₂ that is of normal loudness suggests first-degree A-V block.

3. Which situations can be diagnosed by hearing the effect of a changing P–R interval on the M₁?

ANS: Any **atrioventricular (AV) dissociation**, as in complete AV block or some ventricular tachycardias. (If the ventricular tachycardia has retro-grade VA conduction into the atria, there will be no AV dissociation.)

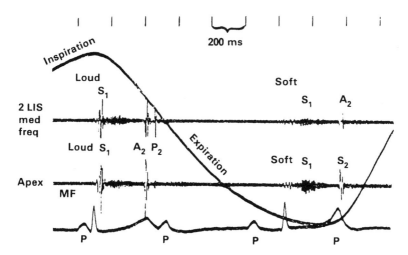

This medium-frequency (MF) phonocardiogram is from a patient with complete AV block, i.e., the P waves and QRS complexes are independent, thus causing the P–R intervals to vary. Note the loud S₁ after the short P–R (first one) and the soft one after the long P–R both at the apex and second left interspace (2 LIS).

Note: Type 1 second-degree AV block (Wenckebach periods) also has gradu-ally longer P–R intervals until complete AV block occurs and a beat is dropped. The gradually longer P–R interval has been said to cause a softer and softer first sound until a pause occurs. However, if the long-est P–R is very long (e.g., about 360 ms), the valves may reopen owing to continued pulmonary venous return, and so produce a slight increase in loudness. Often, though, the P–R changes are so small that no per-ceptible M_1 changes occur.

4. How does left bundle branch block (LBBB) affect the loudness of the M_1?

   ANS: The onset of LV contraction may be delayed so that the effect of a long P–R interval is produced.

REFERENCES

1. Mills, P G., et al. Echocardiographic and hemodynamic relationships of ejection sounds. *Circulation* 56:430, 1977.
2. Shah, P. M., Kramer, D. H., and Gramiak, R. Influence of the timing of atrial systole on mitral valve closure and on the first heart sound in man. *Am. J. Cardiol.* 26:231, 1970.
3. Leech, G., et al. Mechanism of influence of PR interval on loudness of first heart sound. *Br. Heart J.* 43:138, 1980.

9 The Second Heart Sound (S₂)

PHYSIOLOGY AND NOMENCLATURE FOR THE S₂

1. What produces the normal second heart sound (S_2)?

   ANS: Events associated with closure of the aortic and pulmonary valves.

   Note: Valve "closure" itself probably produces no noise. Echocardiography shows that the sounds occur slightly after the coaptation of the leaflets. Shortly after apposition the sealed cusps are made tense and then vibrate (stretch and recoil) due to the rapid force of aortic or pulmonary artery recoil [1].

2. Which valve normally closes first, the aortic or the pulmonary valve?

   ANS: The aortic valve. (It is crucial to remember this.) The sequence is A, P (i.e., aortic and pulmonary), as in Atlantic and Pacific. The A comes first, as in the alphabet. We shall call the aortic component of the second sound A_2 and the pulmonary component P_2.

3. What is the old meaning of A_2 and P_2 (to which we shall *not* refer in this book)?

   ANS: A_2 used to mean the total S_2 in the traditional "aortic area" (second right interspace). P_2 used to mean the total S_2 in the traditional "pulmonary area" (second left interspace). We now use A_2 to mean only the aortic component of the S_2, and P_2 to mean the pulmonary component of the S_2.

A_2 is the aortic valve closure component of the S_2.
P_2 is the pulmonary valve closure component of the S_2. Note that the S_2 occurs near the end of the T wave of the ECG; i.e., the T wave is a systolic event.

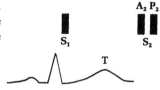

133

EXPLANATION OF NORMAL SPLITTING SEQUENCE OF S₂ ——

1. Draw the ventricular pressure curve and an aortic pressure curve.

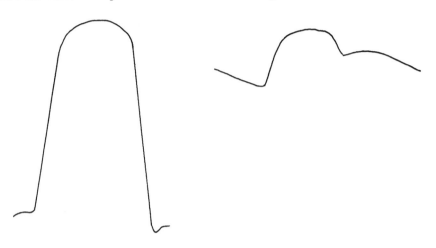

2. Superimpose the aortic pressure curve on the ventricular pressure curve.

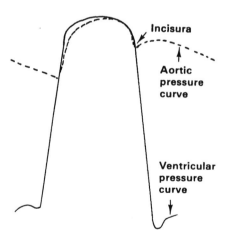

Note that when the LV pressure rise exceeds aortic pressure, the aortic valve will open and produce a single-chamber effect or an "aortoventricle." The point at which ejection is finished and the aortic and LV pressure curves separate is called the incisura and is simultaneous with the aortic second sound, or A₂.

3. At what pressure in the left ventricle (LV) would you expect the aortic valve to open, assuming a normal blood pressure of 120/80 mmHg?

   ANS: When pressure in the LV rises to just above aortic diastolic pressure (about 80 mmHg), the aortic valve will open.

4. After the aortic valve opens, what is the difference in pressure between the LV and the aorta?

    ANS: Almost none. The LV and the aorta are almost a single pressure chamber as soon as the aortic valve opens. (It may be called an "aortoventricle" at this time.) Only in the presence of aortic stenosis (AS) is there a significant pressure difference (gradient) between the aorta and the ventricle.

    Note: In fact, there is normally a slight positive gradient between the LV and the aorta during the first two-thirds to three-fourths of systole. It has been called an impulse gradient.

5. What do we call the notch on the carotid or aortic pressure tracing that occurs roughly at the time of aortic valve closure? How is it related to the heart sounds?

    ANS: In the external carotid tracing taken by putting a pressure-sensitive pickup on the neck, it is called the *dicrotic notch*. In aortic pressure tracings, it is called the *incisura*. The incisura is simultaneous with the A_2 if aortic root pressure tracings are used for timing.

6. At what pressure does the A_2 occur, i.e., does it occur at aortic systolic, diastolic, or some intermediate pressure?

    ANS: The aortic valve closes when the force of ventricular ejection decreases, and the peripheral resistance plus the elastic recoil of the expanded aorta overcomes the decreasing pressure in the LV. This occurs at just below aortic systolic pressure (e.g., if the systolic pressure in the aorta is 120 mmHg, the A_2 probably occurs at a pressure of about 110 mmHg).

    Note: The pulmonary artery pressure tracing also has a dicrotic notch or incisura where the P_2 occurs. The normal pulmonary artery pressure is about 25/10 mmHg.

7. If the aortic valve closes at a pressure of about 100 mmHg, and the pulmonary valve closes at about 20 mmHg, why will aortic closure occur first?

    ANS: The second heart sounds occur simultaneously with the incisuras of the pulmonary artery and aorta. The timing of the incisuras, in turn, has been shown to be related to the impedance to flow. For example, the less the arteriolar resistance and elastic recoil of the pulmonary arteries, the longer will forward flow continue and the later will the incisura occur on the pressure curve of the pulmonary artery. The pulmonary vascular resistance is about a tenth of that of the systemic resistance and the elastic recoil of the normal pulmonary artery is probably less than that of the aorta. Therefore, forward flow continues longer in the pulmonary circuit than in the aortic circuit after their respective pressure crossovers. This causes the pulmonary pressure and closure sound (P_2) to occur later than the aortic incisura and A_2.

PHYSIOLOGY OF THE NORMALLY MOVING SPLIT_____

1. Does the normal split of the S_2 widen on inspiration or expiration?

    ANS: It widens on inspiration, so that the A_2P_2 becomes an A_2–P_2.

2. Does the split movement of the S_2 occur because of the movement of the A_2 or the movement of the P_2?

    ANS: Both. The P_2 moves out, away from the A_2, and the A_2 moves inward, away from the P_2.

3. Which component moves more, the A_2 or the P_2?

    ANS: The P_2.

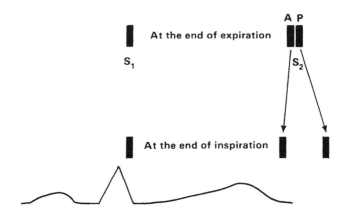

The P_2 outward movement contributes more to the inspiratory widening of the S_2 than does the inward movement of the A_2.

4. Why does the P_2 occur later with inspiration?

    ANS: a. The right ventricle (RV) becomes larger with inspiration because inspiration lowers the intrathoracic pressure (makes it more negative), and this acts to draw more blood from the superior and inferior venae cavae into the right side of the heart. The lungs act as a bellows, i.e., when they expand, they function like a suction apparatus, which sucks blood from the inferior and superior venae cavae into the right atrium and ventricle. This increased RV volume on inspiration delays pulmonary closure because when a ventricle increases its volume and has only one outlet for systole, it takes longer to eject that extra volume.

b. On inspiration the pulmonary impedance falls because the capacitance of the pulmonary vasculature is increased. This also contributes to the delay in pulmonary valve closure.

5. Why does the A_2 occur earlier with inspiration?

ANS: Because the LV becomes smaller with inspiration. This occurs because inspiration, by enlarging the chest volume, also enlarges the vascular capacity of the lungs so much that they cannot compensate by drawing enough blood from the RV. In other words, the lungs do not fill from the RV in proportion to their increase in blood space potential during inspiration. This excessive increase in lung capacity withholds some blood from the LV.

Note: Maximum widening of the split A_2–P_2 occurs at the peak of inspiration. Maximum narrowing occurs during mid-expiration.

6. Does the normally moving split phenomenon (i.e., widening on inspiration and narrowing on expiration) refer to (a) held expiration and inspiration or to moving respiration, and to (b) deep or normal respiration?

ANS: a. It refers to moving respiration.
b. It refers to normal depth of respiration.

Note: a. A split S_2 at end-expiration is so rare after age 50 that it should be considered abnormal.
b. It is easier to hear the normally split S_2 in the upright position because upright posture exaggerates most respiratory effects.

LOUDNESS OF THE COMPONENTS OF S₂ ————————————

The Psychology and Physics of Loudness

1. Is the greatest amplitude or loudness of the components of the S_2 in the low-, medium-, or high-frequency range?

ANS: In the low- and medium-frequency range.

2. Since the bell is best for bringing out low and medium frequencies, why is it usually better to listen to the splitting of the S_2 with the diaphragm?

ANS: The diaphragm separates the two components of the split better. Soft, high-frequency components are masked by louder and longer low and medium frequencies unless they are markedly separated in pitch and width. Because the diaphragm damps out the louder low- and medium-frequencies, which reverberate around the high ones, volume is sacrificed for clarity in separating the components. Therefore, if one of the components of S_2 is very soft, the bell may actually bring it out better.

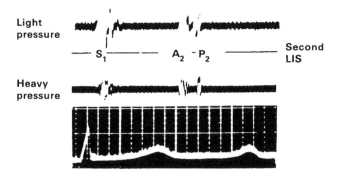

With light pressure, the low and medium frequencies domi-
nate and cause the split sounds (about 50 ms [0.05 s] apart) to
run together. Heavy pressure, by turning the skin into a diaphragm, attenuates the reverberations of the low and medium
frequencies and helps to separate the components of the split.

3. Why does more volume going through the valve make an A_2 or P_2 loud?

   ANS: If the aortic or pulmonary artery root is distended by an increased volume, the distended aorta or pulmonary artery beyond the valve has a
   greater recoil velocity, which closes the valve with more energy.

Sites of A_2 and P_2 Loudness

1. What is wrong with using the expression "A_2 is louder than P_2," or vice versa?

   ANS: If by A_2 is meant the entire second sound in the second right interspace
   and by P_2 is meant the entire second sound in the second left interspace
   (as was true before 1960), then it has no meaning. If it refers to individual components of a split second sound, then "A_2 is louder than P_2,"
   or vice versa may have meaning.

2. Which component of the S_2 is best heard in normal subjects at the second left
   interspace (formerly called the "pulmonary area")? What is the clinical significance of this?

   ANS: Not only is the A_2 louder than the P_2 in the second left interspace in
   70% of normal subjects in all age groups, but also in subjects over age
   20 *the A2 is always normally louder than the P2 in the second left
   interspace* [2]. This, together with the fact that the P_2 is often best heard
   in the third or fourth left interspace, rules out the second left interspace
   as truly a pulmonary area. Because this term is misleading, we encour-
   age use of the term *second left interspace* instead.

3. Where is the A_2 normally heard on the chest wall?

   ANS: Anywhere that one would normally listen for heart sounds.

4. Where is the P_2 normally heard on the chest wall?

    ANS: In adults the P_2 is normally heard all along the left sternal border, often only a few centimeters to the left of the sternum. In infants and young children and in young adults with a thin chest wall and a narrow antero-posterior chest diameter, it may also be heard at the apex.

    Note: This implies that if the P_2 (split S_2) is also heard to the right of the sternum or at the apex in a thick-chested adult, the P_2 is probably louder than normal. When the P_2 is heard unexpectedly at the apex, you will usually find that the RV is enlarged and the apex beat is not due to the LV but entirely to the RV. Thus, in **atrial septal defects** (ASDs) it is expected that the large RV will make the P_2 audible at the apex, even though there may be no pulmonary hypertension.

5. Where is the splitting of the S_2 most often appreciated on the chest wall?

    ANS: At the second or third left interspace parasternally.

    Note: In cyanotic **tetralogy of Fallot**, the S_2 is usually single and consists entirely of the A_2 because the P_2 is attenuated by

        a. A deformed pulmonary valve when there is valvular stenosis.

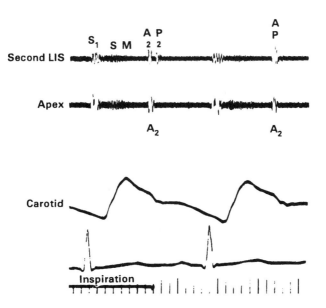

This simultaneous carotid pulse tracing and phonocardiogram is from a normal 16-year-old with a normal split of S_2 on inspiration. Note that (1) only the A_2 would be audible at the apex, and (2) the A_2 has a greater amplitude than the P_2 at the second left interspace (Second LIS).

Boldface type indicates that the term is explained in the glossary.

b. The anterior placement of the aorta relative to a posteriorly placed pulmonary artery.

c. S_2 splitting is best heard to the right of the sternum in dextrocardia and transposition of the great vessels.

6. Where is the aortic component of the S_2 usually heard best in normal subjects of all ages?

ANS: At the second and third left interspaces, probably because the aortic valve is situated behind the sternum, close to this area. This fact further denies that the second right interspace should be called the aortic area, as it is in most of the auscultation literature.

Causes of a Loud A_2 or P_2

1. What conditions tend to make the aortic component of the second sound louder than normal?

ANS: a. Conditions that raise aortic systolic pressure, e.g., systemic hypertension, which occasionally produces a drumlike sound or "tambour" S_2. A tambour is a small drum that is covered only on one side. The tambour effect may persist even after the blood pressure has been lowered to normal by medication.

b. Conditions that produce a hyperkinetic systemic circulation, e.g., youth, or thyrotoxicosis.

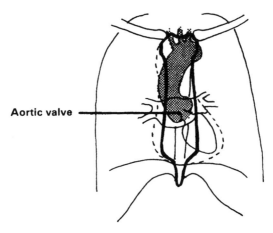

Aortic valve

The root of the aorta with its aortic valve is behind the middle of the sternum.

Note: The loudness of the aortic closure depends on the recoil of the aorta and on ventricular performance [3]. It follows, then, that a hypertensive patient in heart failure may not have a loud A$_2$.

2. What conditions, besides a thin chest wall and pulmonary hypertension, tend to make the P$_2$ louder than normal?

ANS: Conditions that produce increased blood flow into the pulmonary artery, as in ASD or VSD.

3. Why does the A$_2$ tend to be loud when the heart is hyperactive as in thyrotoxicosis and aortic regurgitation (AR)?

ANS: The intensity of the A$_2$ is increased if the aortic valve closes when the aorta is energetically recoiling from the violent stretch due to the increased volume flung into it during systole.

Note: With severe AR the A$_2$ may be soft, presumably because of the absence of adequate valve substance to cause a sudden deceleration of forward flow.

4. How does inspiration affect the loudness of each component of the S$_2$?

ANS: The P$_2$ commonly becomes louder because extra blood in the pulmonary artery on inspiration causes more energetic elastic recoil. The A$_2$, on the other hand, becomes softer because inspiration decreases the volume ejected into the aorta and also places the aorta farther from the stethoscope.

Note: All sounds tend to become softer on inspiration if you listen over the upper chest, where excess lung space is interposed between the stethoscope and the heart on inspiration.

Causes of a Softer A$_2$ or P$_2$

1. What can make either the A$_2$ or the P$_2$ softer than normal besides the effect of an abnormal chest shape and thickness?

ANS: a. Conditions that lower systolic pressure.
b. Conditions that decrease the elastic recoil power of the aortic or pulmonary roots, such as poor myocardial contractility.
c. Conditions that stiffen the semilunar valve (e.g., calcification, sclerosis, or fusion of the cusps, as in AS or pulmonary stenosis [PS]).

Note: In PS the pulmonary valve is thick and leathery. This not only makes the P$_2$ soft but also adds to its lateness, because the RV pressure must drop considerably below the pulmonary artery pressure before it can move the relatively immobile valve.

Relative Loudness, Pitch, and Duration of the S_1 and S_2

1. When is it difficult to distinguish an S_1 from S_2 by stethoscope alone?

   ANS: When systole almost equals diastole in duration. This is called a "ticktack" rhythm (like the ticking of a clock) or embryocardia (like the fetal heart sounds).

2. What causes ticktack rhythm?

   ANS: Anything that shortens diastole more than it does systole, as in tachycardia. As the heart rate increases, both systole and diastole are shortened, but diastole is shortened relatively more than systole.

   Note: a. The heart rate in the first year of life may be as high as 190, and in the second year up to 160. In the fourth year it can normally be 130. Even at the time of puberty it may be as high as 100 normally. This in the adult would be called a tachycardia.

   b. Severe AR may also produce a ticktack rhythm because it can prolong systole in relation to diastole.

3. How may the relative loudness of the S_1 and S_2 help to distinguish one from the other?

   ANS: The S_2 is normally louder than the S_1 at the second right or left interspace (i.e., at the base of the heart), possibly because this is where the aortic and pulmonary valve structures are closest to the chest wall. At the apex the S_1 is usually louder than the S_2.

   Note: The apex area is not as reliable as the base for distinguishing an S_1 from an S_2 by loudness, because with a long P–R interval or with myocardial damage, the S_1 may be very soft.

4. How can you tell at the bedside which heart sound is the S_2 when relative loudness is of no help?

   ANS: a. The S_2 is higher in pitch as well as sharper and shorter than the S_1 because it is usually single on expiration. The S_1 is relatively rough because of its three components and its dominant low and medium frequencies. This is implied by the term "lub-dup," which is often used to mimic the sound of the S_1–S_2.

   b. Palpate the carotid while listening with the stethoscope. The S_1 will be heard just before the carotid impulse is felt. The carotid has the same relationship to the S_1 as an early systolic murmur (i.e., if we use the letter C to represent the carotid impulse, then the rhythm goes "1-C-2, 1-C-2"). This is due to the slight delay between the beginning of ventricular contraction, which produces the S_1, and the arrival of the carotid impulse in the neck.

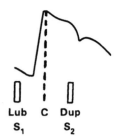

Lub   C   Dup
S$_1$ S$_2$

The tap of the carotid pulse on your fingers is felt *after* and not *with* the first heart sound.

c. Place the stethoscope or a finger over the apex beat, and note the outward impulse that occurs during systole. It should bulge outward with or just after the S$_1$. The stethoscope itself will rise during systole, and this will tell you which sound is the S$_1$. The S$_1$ will appear to "produce" the rise in apical impulse.

THE WIDELY SPLIT S$_2$

1. What is meant by a wide split of the S$_2$?

    ANS: A persistent split that widens on inspiration to at least 60 ms (0.06 s). (Say "pa-da" as quickly as possible for 60 ms.)

    Note: The concept of wide and narrow splitting is best understood if you practice the vocal imitation of splitting widths as follows: A normal narrow split on inspiration is 30–40 ms (0.03–0.04 s). Imitate this by rolling the tongue, as in the Spanish *dr* or *tr*. For a slightly wider split of 50–60 ms (0.05–0.06 s) say "pa-da" quickly. For a wide split of 70–80 ms (0.07–0.08 s) say "pa-ta" quickly. Articulate both the *p* and the *t* sharply. For a very wide split of 90–100 ms (0.09–0.10 s) say "pa-pa" as quickly as possible.

2. What conditions can cause wide splitting of the S$_2$ as a result of a delay in pulmonary valve closure?

    ANS: Delays of P$_2$ are caused by the following:

    a. Conditions that cause electrical delay of activation of the RV (e.g., right bundle branch block [RBBB]).
    b. Conditions that cause an increased volume in the RV in comparison with the LV (e.g., ASD).
    c. Conditions that cause a gradient across the pulmonary valve due to valvular or **infundibular** PS.

    d. Conditions that cause either acute or chronic RV failure, as in massive pulmonary embolism, or in the late stages of **primary pulmonary hypertension**.

Note: a. In massive pulmonary embolism the P_2 may not be accentuated because of the decrease in ejection force due to the increase in afterload.

    b. If the blood volume is increased equally in both ventricles, as in pregnancy or advanced renal failure, the $Q–P_2$ is prolonged more than is the $Q–A_2$ interval so that the split S_2 tends to be wide.

THE $A_2–P_2$ IN PULMONARY STENOSIS

1. Why will a stenotic RV outflow tract or valve cause a delay of the P_2?

    ANS: In PS, RV pressure rises to a much higher level than does pulmonary artery pressure. Thus it takes an extra-long time for the RV pressure to drop to the closing pressure of the pulmonary artery valve. Also, RV pressure will have to fall farther below the pulmonary artery pressure before it can move the rigid valve into the closed position. Furthermore, if there is poststenotic dilatation, the increased pulmonary capacitance plus the poor elastic recoil will increase the delay in P_2.

    Note: A long systolic murmur that continues into or through the A_2 along the left sternal border can obscure the widely split S_2. You can easily tell if the murmur is obscuring an A_2 by exploring the split S_2 away from the maximal murmur area.

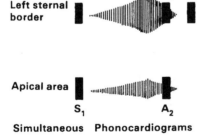

At the apex, the easily recorded A_2 may be heard despite the murmur, which is much softer in that area.

Simultaneous   Phonocardiograms

2. How can the $A_2–P_2$ interval tell you the probable RV pressure in PS?

    ANS: In general, the more severe the obstruction and the higher the RV pressure, the longer the $A_2–P_2$ interval.

The Fixed Split of S₂

1. What can cause a fixed or relatively fixed split of the S₂?

    ANS: a. An ASD.

    b. Heart failure, because it prevents the ventricles from responding to changes in volume and pressure [4]. The heart in failure is relatively insensitive to changes in filling pressure; for example, a rise in the LV end-diastolic pressure of a few millimeters of mercury in the normal ventricle can almost double cardiac output. In the failing ventricle the output rises only slightly or not at all.

    Note: A relatively fixed split in the supine position is a variation of normal in children and young men. The reason is unknown. It will not be fixed in the sitting position.

2. Why is the S₂ split in ASD relatively fixed?

    ANS: In ASD the LV does not become smaller on inspiration and may even become larger because on inspiration vena caval blood is drawn into the right atrium, whose pressure then rises and thereby decreases the left-to-right shunt. This nonshunted left atrial blood passes instead through the mitral valve into the LV and thus tends to keep LV volume constant during inspiration.

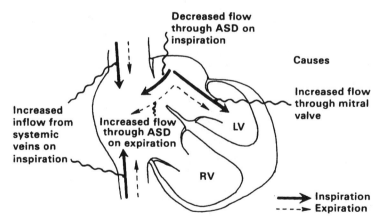

The increased inflow into the right atrium on inspiration (vertical solid arrows) causes a decreased flow through the ASD and thus increased flow through the mitral valve.

3. Does the P₂ move normally with respiration in the presence of an ASD?

    ANS: With normal respiration the P₂ moves only slightly. But with deep inspiration the P₂ in patients with ASD can move almost normally.

4. How does the A_2 move in ASD?

    ANS: Either not at all or slightly toward the P_2 on inspiration. This latter movement is actually a reversal of normal movement.

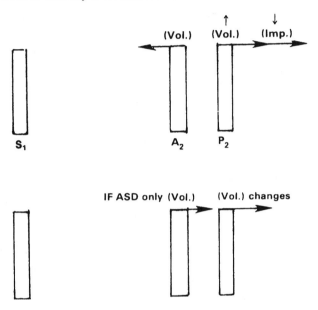

On inspiration the P_2 is shown to be moving to the right away from the S_1 by two mechanisms, the increased volume in the RV and the decreased impedance of the pulmonary circuit. The A_2 is shown moving to the left (toward the S_1) by only one mechanism, the decreased volume in the LV. In ASDs the P_2 moves with inspiration due only to its increased volume, because there is no significant impedance effect when the lung vessels are overfilled because of the shunt flow. The A_2 may either not move at all with inspiration or actually move in the same direction as the P_2.

ASDs WITH NARROW SPLITS

1. How common is a narrow split of the S_2 with ASDs?

    ANS: Although ASDs are noted for their wide splits, the majority of adults with ASDs do not have a split of more than 60 ms, which is as short as it takes to say "pa-da" as quickly as possible.

    Note: a. A narrow split on inspiration that remains split on expiration, especially during sitting or standing, is an excellent sign of a relatively fixed split, because if a split is narrow on inspiration, it should close on expiration, especially in the sitting or standing position.

b. The degree of splitting seems to be related to the degree of dilatation of the pulmonary artery. This may explain why closure of the
ASD in older adults does not narrow the split.

DIFFERENTIAL DIAGNOSIS OF THE FIXED SPLIT _____

1. What may mimic a wide fixed split of the S$_2$?

   ANS: a. The A$_2$ followed by an opening snap.
   b. A very wide split in which normal movements of the A$_2$–P$_2$ are difficult to perceive by auscultation.

2. Why does the split S$_2$ in the normal subject tend to narrow on sitting or standing?

   ANS: This happens because when both ventricles receive less blood (due to
   pooling in the abdomen and the legs), the RV responds by ejecting its
   blood relatively faster than does the LV [5]. The RV responds more to
   changes in filling pressure than does the LV.

3. What happens to the splitting of the S$_2$ after a Valsalva maneuver during the
   period immediately following release and then a few seconds afterward? How
   can you use this maneuver to detect the presence of an ASD?

   ANS: In normal subjects the split widens immediately on release. This occurs
   because the Valsalva maneuver dams up venous blood behind the RV.
   On release of this dammed-up blood, there is extra filling in the RV for
   a few beats, in contrast to the LV, which actually contains less blood for
   a few beats because the lungs have been partially emptied.

   A few seconds after the release of the strain, the split S$_2$ becomes
   very narrow or single because the dammed-up blood now reaches the
   LV, pushing a comparatively greater volume into the LV than into the
   RV for a few beats.

   In patients with ASDs, however, the atria act almost as a single
   chamber so that any rise in right atrial pressure is also reflected in a rise
   in left atrial pressure. Thus, on release of the Valsalva maneuver, any
   increased venous blood that rushes into the RV will also cause more
   blood to enter the LV, and there will be only slight immediate widening
   and no delayed narrowing of the S$_2$.

   Note: You can overcome difficulties in a patient's understanding of how to
   perform a Valsalva maneuver by asking the patient to push against
   your hand while it is pressed against the patient's abdomen. Blowing
   a manometer up to 40 mmHg is the ideal method of performing a
   Valsalva maneuver.

4. How can you distinguish the wide, fixed split and loud P_2 of RV failure due to pulmonary hypertension from that of ASD with pulmonary hypertension?

ANS: Exercise will widen the split still further only in RV failure because it delays the P_2, probably because the rise in pulmonary artery pressure with exercise will increase the isovolumic contraction time of the failing RV and leave the isovolumic contraction of the normal LV relatively unchanged.

THE NARROWLY SPLIT S_2

1. List the usual causes of a narrowly split S_2 due to a delayed A_2.

ANS: a. Conditions that cause electrical delay of LV conduction, such as left bundle branch block (LBBB).

b. Conditions that increase the volume of the LV but without an extra outlet (a VSD or mitral regurgitation [MR] is an extra outlet), e.g., persistent ductus arteriosus (PDA) and AR.

c. Conditions that cause a significant gradient across the outflow tract of the LV (e.g., AS), so that there is a delay in LV pressure dropping below aortic pressure.

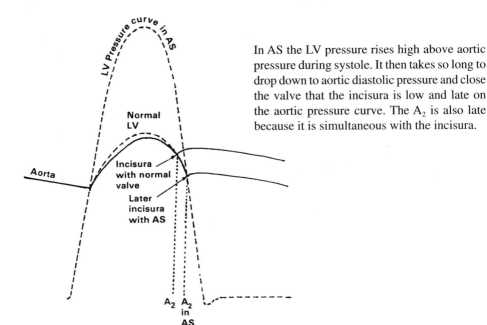

In AS the LV pressure rises high above aortic pressure during systole. It then takes so long to drop down to aortic diastolic pressure and close the valve that the incisura is low and late on the aortic pressure curve. The A_2 is also late because it is simultaneous with the incisura.

2. The S_2 is single on quiet inspiration in about what percentage of normal subjects (a) under age 50 and (b) over age 50?

   ANS: The S_2 is single.

   a. In about 30% of subjects under age 50.
   b. In about 60% of subjects over age 60 [6].

   Note: Prolongation of LV isovolumic contraction time contributes to the delayed A_2 and narrowness of the split S_2 with aging.

3. How can you tell that an S_2 is split on inspiration even if you do not hear two distinct components?

   ANS: If the S_2 is clean and sharp on expiration and becomes impure or rough on inspiration.

4. What kinds of respiration will obscure awareness of whether the split moves besides rapid respiration?

   ANS: a. Too deep an inspiration will interpose too much lung between the stethoscope and the heart, causing one or both of the S_2 components to disappear.
   b. Too shallow an inspiration may not open the S_2 at all.

   Note: If you raise your arm for inspiration and lower it for expiration, you may "conduct" respiration so that there are at least two or three cycles during each phase of respiration. Be certain that the patient does not breathe too deeply.

THE S_2 SPLIT IN PULMONARY HYPERTENSION ⸻

1. What are the three general types of pulmonary hypertension?

   ANS: a. Hyperkinetic pulmonary hypertension, i.e., that due to excess volume flow, as in large left-to-right shunts. The pulmonary arterioles can dilate to accommodate up to three times the normal cardiac output before the pulmonary artery pressure must rise.
   b. Vasoactive pulmonary hypertension, i.e., that due primarily to pulmonary arteriolar constriction, as in response to either hypoxia or to a high left atrial pressure, as in patients with mitral stenosis (MS).
   c. Obstructive pulmonary hypertension, i.e., that due to fixed lumen obliteration, as with pulmonary emboli, or to narrowing, as with the endothelial and medial hypertrophy seen in some ASDs, PDAs, and VSDs with bidirectional shunting (**Eisenmenger reaction**), or with primary pulmonary hypertension.

2. How much obstruction is necessary before an acute pulmonary embolism can produce wide, relatively fixed splitting of the S_2?

   ANS: Almost the entire pulmonary tree on both sides must be obstructed. If, however, pulmonary hypertension is already present due to previous disease, a further embolus to one branch may cause wide, fixed splitting.

3. Why does the S_2 of a VSD with an Eisenmenger reaction become single?

   ANS: This occurs because only a large VSD could produce an Eisenmenger reaction, and such a large communication between the ventricles tends to make them function as a single chamber.

4. How does the S_2 differ among the three different levels of Eisenmenger syndromes, i.e., VSD, ASD, and PDA?

   ANS: In VSDs the S_2 is single; in ASDs it is split and fixed (often widely split); in PDAs it is normally or narrowly split and when split, it moves normally with respiration.

THE REVERSED OR PARADOXICALLY SPLIT S_2 ————————

Physiology and Etiologies

1. What is meant by a reversed or paradoxical split of the S_2?

   ANS: This is a split in which the order of components is P_2A_2 instead of the normal A_2P_2.

2. Can too early a P_2 cause a reversed split?

   ANS: A reversed split is nearly always caused by a delayed A_2.

3. What can delay the A_2 enough to cause a paradoxical splitting?

   ANS: a. Conduction defects that delay depolarization of the LV, such as complete LBBB and some types of Wolff-Parkinson-White (W-P-W) preexcitation that imitate LBBB.

   Note: The type of W-P-W preexcitation that acts like LBBB is one in which the initial conduction passes to the RV muscle first. This is known as type B, in which the QRS and delta wave in V_1 point predominantly posteriorly (i.e., they are predominantly negative).

   b. Aortic stenosis with a marked systolic gradient across the aortic valve, causing a delay in the fall of LV pressure to below aortic pressure.

   c. Hypertension plus myocardial damage.

4. What causes the widest reversed split?

   ANS: Complete LBBB (i.e., with a QRS of 120 ms [0.12 s] or longer). This is also the most common cause of a reversed split and the only one that is easily recognized by the noncardiologist.

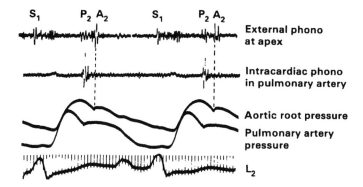

S$_1$ P$_2$ A$_2$ S$_1$ P$_2$ A$_2$

External phono at apex

Intracardiac phono in pulmonary artery

Aortic root pressure

Pulmonary artery pressure

L$_2$

These simultaneous intra-arterial and phonocardiogram tracings are from a 59-year-old man in heart failure due to an idiopathic cardiomyopathy. Because of LBBB, the incisura of the pulmonary artery and its simultaneous P$_2$ comes before the aortic incisura and its simultaneous A$_2$. (His pulmonary artery systolic pressure was 35 mmHg; his LV pressure, 120 mmHg; and his cardiac index, 2.4). These are catheter-tip electromanometer tracings, so that there are no tubing delays.

5. What is the significance of expiratory splitting of the S$_2$?

   ANS: Expiratory splitting indicates either a wide split, a fixed split, or a paradoxical split.

6. What causes the most common confusion with paradoxical splitting of S$_2$?

   ANS: An S$_2$-opening snap. (This is discussed in detail in Chapter 10.)

7. How can S$_2$ splitting differentiate a PAC from a PVC?

   ANS: If a premature beat has narrow or no splitting of S$_2$, it is probably supraventricular.

Eliciting and Recognizing Reversed Splits

1. What should make you suspect paradoxical or reversed splitting?

   ANS: A split that widens on expiration and narrows on inspiration implies that the P$_2$ comes first.

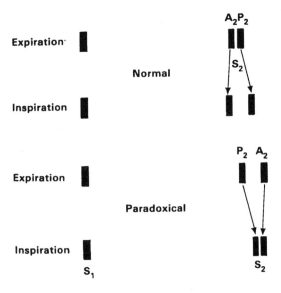

If the split narrows on inspiration, the P_2 must come first, and the split S_2 is reversed.

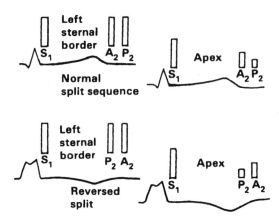

If the split is fixed at the left sternal border, it may be difficult to tell whether it has a normal or paradoxical sequence. Toward the apex, the component that becomes relatively softer must be the P_2.

2. How can you confirm by auscultation that a wide split is reversed when the respiratory movements are so erratic that the respiratory changes cannot be used?

    ANS: a. At the apex the A$_2$ is either the only sound heard, or it is the loudest component of the S$_2$ if both are heard there. Therefore, you should gradually move your stethoscope from the left sternal border toward the apex as you listen to the split second sound. The S$_2$ component that either disappears or becomes softer at the apex will be the P$_2$. If you hear the first component becoming softer or disappearing in relation to the second component, then the order is P$_2$A$_2$. Since the A$_2$ is usually the only component of S$_2$ heard at the second right interspace, the same maneuver can be used by gradually shifting your chest piece toward the second right interspace. If the split is also heard in the second right interspace, which is part of the aortic area, and the second component is louder than the first, then you know that you are listening to P$_2$A$_2$ or a reversed split.

    b. The component that increases in loudness with inspiration is the P$_2$.

REFERENCES

1. Laniado, S., et al. Hemodynamic correlates of the normal aortic valve echogram. A study of sound, flow, and motion. *Circulation* 54:729, 1976.
2. Sainani. G. S., and Luisada, A.A. "Mapping" the precordium. *Am. J. Cardiol.* 19:788, 1967.
3. Stein, P. D., Sabbah, H. N., and Blick, E. F. Dependence of the intensity of the aortic closure sound upon the rate of ventricular diastolic relaxation and ventricular performance. *Am. J. Cardiol.* 39:287, 1977.
4. Perloff, J. K., and Harvey, W. P. Mechanisms of fixed splitting of the second heart sound. *Circulation* 18:998, 1958.
5. Moss, W. G., and Johnson, F. Differential effects of stretch upon the stroke volumes of the right and left ventricles. *Am. J. Physiol.* 139:52, 1943.
6. Adolph, R. J., and Fowler, N. O. The second heart sound: A screening test for heart disease. *Mod. Concepts Cardiovasc. Dis.* 39:91, 1970.

10 The Opening Snap

MECHANISM AND TIMING

1. Draw a simultaneous normal left ventricular (LV) and left atrial (LA) pressure curve. At what point on the curve does the mitral valve open?

    ANS: The mitral valve opens when LV pressure drops below LA pressure. The normal peak LA pressure is about 10 mmHg. Therefore, when LV pressure drops to about 9 mmHg, the mitral valve should open.

    Note: LV early expansion has an active suction effect related to the degree of cardiac function or inotropism.

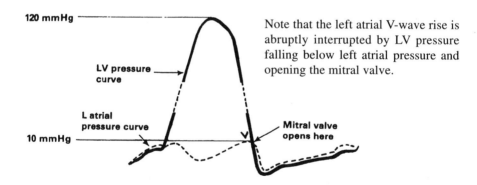

120 mmHg

LV pressure curve

L atrial pressure curve

10 mmHg

Mitral valve opens here

Note that the left atrial V-wave rise is abruptly interrupted by LV pressure falling below left atrial pressure and opening the mitral valve.

2. Draw an LV, LA, and simultaneous aortic pressure curve. Which left-sided event produces a sound just before the mitral valve opens? (See p. 156)

    ANS: Closure of the aortic valve produces the A_2 about 100 ms (0.10 s) before the mitral valve opens. This 100-ms interval takes about as long as it takes to say "pa-pa" as quickly as possible.

3. What is usually necessary before the opening of the mitral valve becomes audible?

    ANS: At least some mitral stenosis (MS), which is due primarily to fibrous thickening and often to calcification of the margins of the mitral leaflets, especially the large anterior leaflet. The mitral valve belly may act like a sail that billows downward into a dome in diastole as the LV attempts to "suck" LA blood into the LV cavity. This sudden diastolic doming caused the anterior leaflet to bulge downward with a snap.

Note: Excessive flow through the mitral valve in early diastole as in VSD, MR, and thyrotoxicosis can also cause an opening snap.

4. Why is the audible opening of the mitral valve called an opening snap (OS)?

   ANS: Because most of the time the sound is a short, high-frequency, crisp crack, click, or snap.

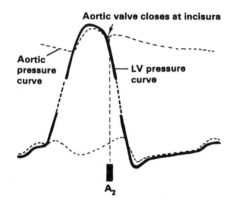

Aortic valve closes at incisura

Aortic pressure curve

LV pressure curve

A_2

The A_2 is simultaneous with the aortic valve incisura and occurs shortly before the LV pressure drops below left atrial pressure, to open the mitral valve. The interval between the aortic valve closure (A_2) and the opening of the mitral valve is the isovolumic relaxation time.

5. Why must it be the anterior leaflet that is responsible for the OS of MS?

   ANS: The anterior leaflet is three times broader than the posterior leaflet.

6. What do we call the interval between the closing of the aortic valve and the opening of the mitral valve?

   ANS: The **isovolumic relaxation** period.

7. What is the auscultatory term for the isovolumic relaxation interval between the aortic closure sound and the OS sound?

   ANS: The A_2–OS interval, or simply the 2–OS interval.

RELATION BETWEEN THE 2–OS INTERVAL AND THE SEVERITY OF MITRAL STENOSIS _____

1. What are the major factors controlling the duration of isovolumic relaxation, or the 2–OS interval?

   ANS: a. The pressure at which the aortic valve closes (near systolic pressure).
   b. The pressure in the LA at the time the mitral valve opens.

2. What is the relationship between the degree of MS and the height of the V wave in the LA?

   ANS: The greater the stenosis, the greater the obstruction to flow and thus the slower and more incomplete is the emptying of the LA. Therefore, the greater the MS, the higher is the V wave.

   Note: This will be clear only if you recall that the V wave is built up during ventricular systole when the mitral valve is closed. If the LA did not empty well in diastole due to MS, the V wave will start to build up from an already high pressure.

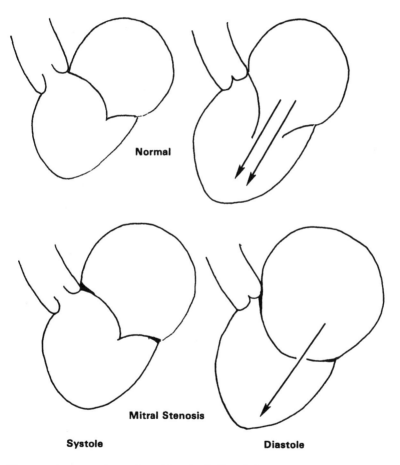

Normal

Mitral Stenosis

Systole   Diastole

The opening snap is produced by the belly of the stenotic anterior leaflet bulging or doming downward with a jerk to produce a clicking or snapping sound. The anterior leaflet, therefore, must also close with a snap as it domes upward. The posterior leaflet has too short a ring-to-free edge distance to produce a "belly snap."

3. Does a high left atrial pressure make the 2–OS interval shorter or longer? Why?

   ANS: Shorter, because the LV pressure does not have to fall so far to open the mitral valve after closure of the aortic valve, or A_2.

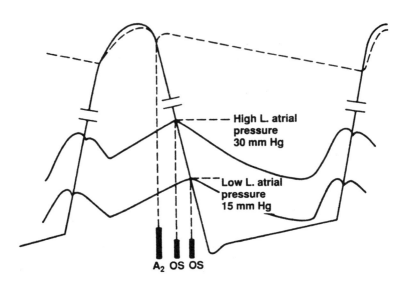

A_2 OS OS

Note that the distance between the A_2 and the OS is shorter with the higher left atrial pressure.

4. List the causes of a late OS aside from a mild degree of MS or a heavily calcified mitral valve.

   ANS: a. Poor myocardial function due to either damage or aging. This causes prolongation of the isovolumic relaxation time. (Isovolumic relaxation time also increases strikingly with age.)

   b. Aortic regurgitation (AR). This is presumably due to the AR jet striking the underbelly of the anterior mitral leaflet and preventing rapid downward excursion of the valve belly. (AR may even eliminate an OS.)

   c. High aortic pressure. If the aortic valve closes at a high pressure, more time will be required for the LV pressure to drop below LA pressure to open the mitral valve and create the OS.

5. Which is more reliable in predicting the degree of MS, a narrow 2–OS interval or a wide one? Why?

   ANS: A narrow 2–OS is more reliable because there is not much besides tight MS or a tachycardia that can narrow a 2–OS interval, whereas there are at least five causes besides mild MS for a wide 2–OS.

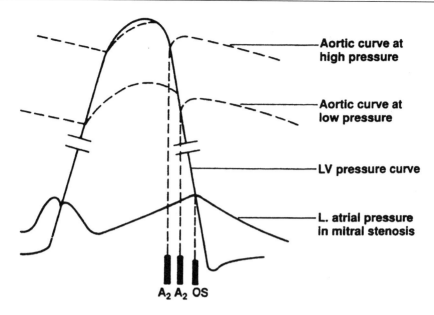

Note that the higher the aortic pressure the longer the A_2-OS interval.

6. Without a phonocardiograph, how can you estimate the width of the 2–OS interval?

   ANS: a. If you say "pa-pa" as quickly as possible, you will be separating the sounds by about 100 ms (0.01 s). This is close to the widest possible 2–OS interval.

   b. If you say "pa-da" as quickly as possible, you should be able to separate the sounds by about 50–70 ms (0.05–.07 s). This is a narrow 2–OS and suggests moderate to tight MS.

THE LOUDNESS OF THE OPENING SNAP

1. Other than an obese or emphysematous chest and AR, what can cause a soft or absent OS despite significant MS?

   ANS: a. The mitral valve may be too calcified for the bellies to snap to their maximal open position. (The S_1 may still be loud.)

   b. Extremely low flow due to exceptional severity of the stenosis, secondary pulmonary hypertension, concomitant aortic or tricuspid valve disease, or myocardial dysfunction.

2. How often does a mitral commissurotomy eliminate the OS?

   ANS: Probably in not more than half the cases.

Note: Normally, a porcine valve may produce a soft OS in two-thirds of patients. The presence or absence of an OS reveals nothing about porcine valve malfunction [1].

HOW TO TELL AN A_2-P_2 FROM AN A_2-OS

Similarities Between a P_2 and the OS

1. Where on the chest wall is the OS usually best heard?

   ANS: An OS is usually best heard between the apex and the left sternal border or at the left sternal border. This is where a P_2 may also be best heard.

2. How does the range of a 2–OS interval differ from that of an A_2-P_2 interval?

   ANS: They do not differ much.

Differences Between the A_2-P_2 and the 2–OS

1. When is an OS louder or as loud at the apex as it is at the left sternal border?

   ANS: As a rule, this occurs only when the LV is dilated, or if a rib has been removed in previous heart surgery. A P_2 is never as loud or louder at the apex than at the left sternal border.

   OS vs P_2 Rule No. 1:
   If the second component of a split S2 is louder or as loud at the apex as at the left sternal border, it is probably an OS.

2. How does the effect of respiration affect the loudness of the P_2 differently from that of the OS?

   ANS: Inspiration makes the P_2 louder (more blood is drawn into the right side of the heart with inspiration) and the OS softer (blood is withheld from the left atrium on inspiration so that less blood flows through the mitral valve).

   OS vs P_2 Rule No. 2:
   If the second component of an S2 split becomes softer on inspiration at the left lower sternal border (in the absence of LBBB), it is probably a mitral OS.

3. How can you recognize an A_2, P_2, and OS as a triple second sound?

   ANS: A triple S_2 can often be recognized along the left sternal border in MS by listening for a snare-drum effect, a "trill," or the "tongue-rolling" Spanish *rr* effect. The snare-drum triple S_2 is most likely to be heard during inspiration, when the P_2 pulls away from the A_2.

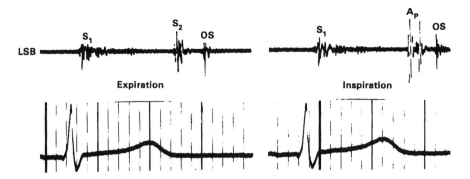

On inspiration, the S_2 split opened up into its A_2 and P_2 components. Together with the OS, a triple second sound is heard that produces a snare-drum effect.

OS vs P_2 Rule No. 3:
   A triple second sound, in which the three sounds are close enough together to sound like a snare drum, implies that an OS is present as the final component.

4. What effect does standing have on the 2–OS interval? Why?

   ANS: It widens it. The pooling of blood in the legs decreases venous return to the left atrium. This lowers the pressure behind the obstructed mitral valve. (For why a low pressure in the LA makes a wide 2–OS interval, see Question 3 above under Relation Between the 2–OS Interval and the Severity of Mitral Stenosis.)

5. What effect does standing have on the A_2-P_2 interval? Why?

   ANS: The A_2-P_2 interval either remains the same or narrows. The reason for this is that although there is a decrease in volume to both ventricles, the right ventricle (RV) responds to the decrease more than does the LV.

OS vs P_2 Rule No. 4:
   If a split second sound becomes wider on standing, its second component is an OS.

6. Why should the presence of an OS imply that the first sound should have a snapping quality?

   ANS: If doming of the valve produced the OS, then it should also make a snapping S_1. In other words, a mitral valve that has an OS usually also has a "closing snap."

OS vs P_2 Rule No. 5:
   If the S2 is very soft, the second component of the S2 is not likely to be an OS.

Summary of Methods of Differentiating an A_2–P_2 from a 2–OS

1. If the second component of a split S_2 is as loud at the apex as at the left sternal border, it is probably an OS.
2. If the second component decreases with inspiration, it is an OS [in the absence of left bundle branch block (LBBB)].
3. If there is a triple second sound at the left sternal border, an OS is present.
4. If the split widens on standing, the second component is an OS.
5. If the S_1 is soft or muffled, the second component of the split S_2 is probably not a mitral OS.

The Tricuspid Opening Snap

1. When will a tricuspid OS be present in the absence of tricuspid stenosis (TS)?

    ANS: a. When a large volume enters the RV by way of the tricuspid valve as with an ASD or anomalous pulmonary venous drainage into the right atrium [2].

              b. With a deformed tricuspid valve, as in the **Ebstein anomaly**.

2. How does the effect of respiration on the mitral and tricuspid opening snaps differ?

    ANS: A tricuspid OS becomes louder on inspiration because more blood flows through the tricuspid valve on inspiration.

REFERENCES _____

1. Raizada, V., et al. Non-invasive evaluation of normally functioning mitral bioprosthesis. *Abstracts, World Congress of Cardiology*, Tokyo, p. 1330, 1978.
2. Tanaka, C., et al. Phonocardiographic findings in adult ASD. *Cardiovasc. Sound Bull.* 5:107, 1975.

Boldface type indicates that the term is explained in the glossary.

11 The Third Heart Sound (S₃)

NOMENCLATURE

1. What are other names for the S_3?

   ANS: The third heart sound, protodiastolic gallop sound, or ventricular gallop.

2. What is misleading about the word *protodiastolic* in describing the S_3?

   ANS: Protodiastolic is used as a synonym for early diastolic, yet the prefix *protos* means not "early" but "first."

3. What is the difference between an S_3 and a ventricular gallop sound?

   ANS: A gallop cannot be one sound. The word *gallop* must refer to a rhythm or cadence made by at least three sounds in succession. A ventricular gallop is the triple rhythm made by the sequence of the S_1, S_2, and S_3. Therefore, the term S_3 is preferable.

4. How has the meaning of the term *gallop rhythm* changed over the decades?

   ANS: This term was originally used to describe any rapid series of three or more sounds in the presence of a tachycardia and heart failure. It included any extra sounds in systole (systolic gallop) as well as diastole. It also eliminated any S_3 with a normal heart rate or without heart failure. Therefore, the term gallop rhythm has changed its meaning, because it now refers to any series of three or more sounds in which the extra sounds occur *only in diastole* and are due to an S_3, an S_4, or both.

TIMING

1. Which left ventricular (LV) hemodynamic events occur in diastole after the S_2 but before the S_3?

   ANS: **Isovolumic relaxation**, and after opening of the mitral valve, early rapid filling of the LV.

2. When does isovolumic relaxation begin and end in the LV?

   ANS: It begins with aortic valve closure and ends with mitral valve opening. As soon as isovolumic relaxation ends and the mitral valve opens, the LV fills rapidly from the left atrium.

Boldface type indicates that the term is explained in the glossary.

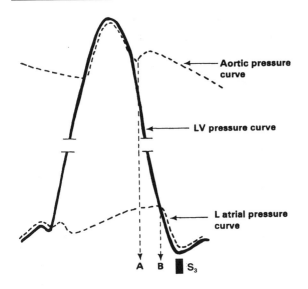

Between point A (aortic valve closure) and point B (mitral valve opening), the volume in the LV is unchanged. This is therefore the isovolumic relaxation period.

3. Does the ventricle fill most rapidly in early, middle, or late diastole?

   ANS: In early diastole. The ventricle has two rates of expansion: an early rapid one and a later slow one. Once the aortic valve opens, the LV expands very rapidly during isovolumic relaxation; even after the mitral valve opens, it continues to expand rapidly during the phase of rapid ventricular filling. From the time the aortic valve closes to make the S_2 to the end of the rapid filling phase when the S_3 occurs is a fairly short period of time of about 120 ms. This can be imitated by saying "two-three" as quickly as possible. At the end of the rapid filling phase, rapid expansion of the ventricle is checked by unknown forces, and the slow expansion phase takes over.

4. What percentage of ventricular filling occurs in the early rapid filling phase of diastole in comparison with the later slow filling phase of diastole?

   ANS: About 80%. After the initial rapid filling, the volume of the ventricle changes very little until atrial contraction squeezes the last 20% of blood into the ventricle.

5. At what point during the rapid filling phase of the LV pressure curve does the S_3 occur?

   ANS: Near the end of the rapid pressure drop in the LV, i.e., near the point at which rapid expansion changes to the slow expansion phase.

   Note: Some rapid filling continues to occur after the S_3.

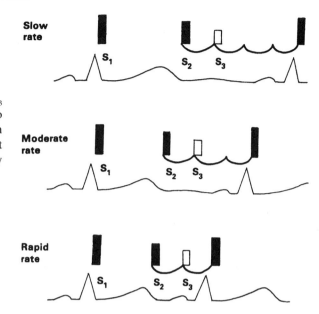

At slow rates (top line) the S_3 is much closer to the S_2 than to the following S_1; i.e., it falls in the first quarter of diastole. At fast rates (bottom line) it may occur in mid-diastole.

6. In what part of diastole does the S_3 usually fall?

    ANS: In the first third in patients with normal heart rates, and in the middle third in those with tachycardias.

MECHANISM OF PRODUCTION

1. How is the S_3 produced?

    ANS: There are two theories: an external and an internal production theory. In the internal production theory the S_3 is due to a sudden "pulling short" of the rapidly expanding ventricle by unknown myocardial forces at the end of the early rapid expansion phase. At the moment of the S_3, the ventricle has suddenly stopped rapid expansion, and the pressure in the ventricle is no longer falling but is relatively stable for about 40 ms, despite continued rapid filling due to the inertia of the blood mass. The S_3 seems to occur at the transition between rapid active and rapid passive ventricular filling when LV pressure rises slightly above left atrial pressure. The continued rapid increase in blood volume in the ventricle at the time of the sudden transition may act as a sudden distending force that causes the sound.

2. How can an external production theory account for the S_3?

> ANS: a. An S_3 often cannot be recorded inside the LV in a patient in whom it can be recorded externally on the chest wall [1].
>
> b. There is no feature of the LV pressure curve that consistently corresponds to the S_3.
>
> c. The apex cardiogram shows a peak of rapid early outward movement at the time of the S_3. When marked, this peak is palpable and is then accompanied by a loud S_3.

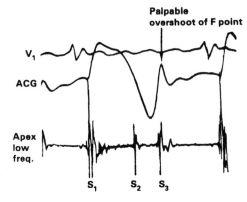

Palpable overshoot of F point

This apex impulse tracing (apex cardiogram) and simultaneous apical phonocardiogram is from a 20-year-old man with heart failure and atrial fibrillation due to a severe idiopathic cardiomyopathy. The pathological S_3 was very loud and was audible everywhere on the chest. It was difficult to say whether it was the overshoot of the rapid filling wave (F point) or the vibration of the S_3 that was palpable.

> d. The loudness of the S_3 is very dependent on how well the apex beat comes out between the ribs and how close the heart is to the chest wall.

3. What is the external production theory for the S_3?

> ANS: During contraction the heart rotates counterclockwise, as viewed from the apex. Its rotation twists the great vessels and stretches the restraining elastic structures that are working to limit its rotation. If the heart rotates with enough energy, its momentum may stretch the restraining structures to such an extent that there is a sudden recoil at the end of its rotation in early diastole. This recoil may throw the heart against the chest wall hard enough to produce a sound.

> *Note*: The internal production theory is more widely accepted.

THE PHYSIOLOGICAL S_3

1. How common is the physiological S_3 in normal subjects?

> ANS: In one study it was recorded on a phonocardiogram near the apex in one-third of normal subjects under age 16 [2]. (This is not to say that it

was audible in all cases in which it was recorded.) It is rarely audible or recordable in normal subjects over age 30.

2. What cardiovascular conditions tend to produce an audible S$_3$ in the normal heart?

ANS: Anything that increases the velocity of ventricular expansion and recoil, such as an increase in flow or sympathetic stimulation, e.g., tachycardia.

3. What does the presence of a physiological S$_3$ tell you about the patient's circulation time?

ANS: It suggests at least a normal **circulation time**. The sympathetic tone and catecholamines that produce the rapid early expansion necessary for the S$_3$ will also increase the cardiac output and accelerate the circulation time.

Note: A venous hum in the neck implies a normal or rapid circulation time, and its presence helps to confirm that the S$_3$ is physiological and is not associated with heart failure. (See Chapter 14 for a method of eliciting a venous hum.)

4. When will a tachycardia produce a loud physiological S$_3$ in a normal patient over age 30?

ANS: There will be a loud S$_3$ if the rapid filling phase of ventricular expansion is augmented by atrial contraction. The gallop rhythm that results is then known as a summation gallop. This will occur when atrial contraction occurs in the early part of diastole, as with a marked tachycardia or with a moderate tachycardia together with a first-degree atrioventricular (AV) block (long P–R interval).

LOUDNESS OF THE S$_3$

1. Which chest piece and degree of stethoscope pressure best brings out the S$_3$?

ANS: The bell, applied with light to moderate pressure so that the low frequencies will not be damped out.

2. What increases the loudness of the S$_3$, inspiration or expiration?

ANS: Either. Expiration can make the S$_3$ louder by squeezing blood out of the lungs into the left atrium and ventricle, and by bringing the stethoscope closer to the heart. Inspiration can make it louder by increasing sympathetic tone to the heart and via a **sinus arrhythmia** speeding up the heart rate and blood flow through the valve.

Note: Either inspiration or expiration can make the S$_3$ louder by causing the apex beat to emerge between the ribs. In some patients the apex beat comes out between the ribs on inspiration, and in others it does so on expiration.

3. Because the proximity of the apex beat to the stethoscope appears to be a factor in intensifying the loudness of the S_3, how can you bring the apex beat closer to the chest wall?

   ANS: By turning the patient into the **left lateral decubitus position**.

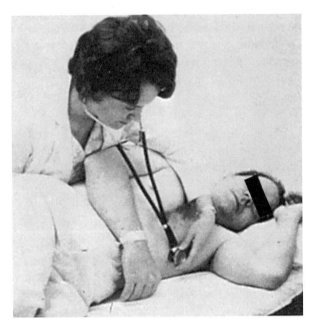

In the left lateral decubitus position shown, the apex of the heart is brought as close to the stethoscope as possible. This is an absolute necessity for hearing a soft S_3, because it is sensitive to proximity.

4. What proof is there that ventricular volume and flow control the audibility of the S_3?

   ANS: a. Conditions that increase the volume of flow make the S_3 louder, i.e., exercise or mitral regurgitation.

   b. Conditions that decrease flow to the heart and decrease ventricular volume cause decreased audibility of the S_3, e.g., standing up, venous tourniquets, or the water-loss effect of diuretics.

   Note: One of the characteristics that is most confusing to the beginner when listening to a soft S_3 is its intermittent audibility, i.e., it waxes and wanes in and out of one's hearing threshold. This probably occurs because its loudness is very sensitive to slight changes in proximity and volume caused by respiration.

THE EXAGGERATED PHYSIOLOGICAL S_3 ————————————

1. List the common shunts and the valvular lesion that may cause excessive flow through the mitral valve, therefore exaggerating or bringing back the physiological S_3.

   ANS: a. The two left-to-right shunts, **ventricular septal defect** (VSD) and **persistent ductus arteriosus** (PDA). (**Atrial septal defects** [ASDs] do not increase flow through the mitral valve.)

   b. An incompetent mitral valve, i.e., mitral regurgitation (MR).

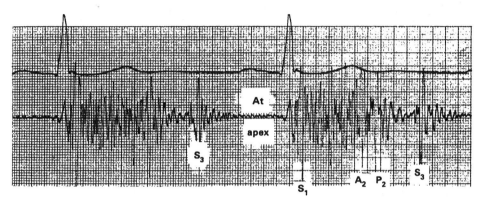

Low-frequency phonocardiogram from a 15-year-old girl with severe rheumatic MR. Besides the loud MR murmur and S_3, note the following: (1) The widely split S_2 (A_2–P_2) expected if moderate to severe MR is present. (2) The P_2 is well heard at the apex and should make you suspect some pulmonary hypertension. The patient's pulmonary artery systolic pressure was 35 mmHg (upper normal is 25 mmHg.)

   Note: Excessive flow through a tricuspid valve does not usually cause a right-sided S_3, i.e., there is no physiological right-sided S_3. The right ventricular (RV] S_3 requires not only a large RV but also a stiff RV and high right atrial pressure. For example, in an uncomplicated ASD with a very large flow through the tricuspid valve, there is usually no S_3. It seems that the RV S_3 occurs only when there is reduced **compliance**. The normal RV is more compliant than the LV and unless it becomes thick because it is also pressure-overloaded, it expands easily to accommodate increased flow.

2. How can the detection of an S_3 tell you whether the pulmonary hypertension in a patient with a VSD or PDA is due to an increased flow (hyperkinetic) or to a fixed irreversible resistance?

   ANS: The presence of a LV S_3 signifies that there is increased flow through the mitral valve and, therefore, also through the pulmonary circuit. The pulmonary hypertension must, therefore, be hyperkinetic and not fixed. This means that surgical closure of the VSD or PDA may lower the pulmonary artery pressure to normal [3].

THE PATHOLOGICAL S_3

1. What are the most common associated cardiac findings with a pathological S_3?

    ANS: A high mean left atrial pressure due to a high V wave, a noncompliant LV, and a large ventricle resulting from a poor **ejection fraction**.

2. What pathological cardiac condition is generally present when an S_3 occurs in the presence of a high left atrial pressure due to a low ejection fraction?

    ANS: A **cardiomyopathy**, most often idiopathic (which is probably viral) or due to extensive ischemic heart disease.

    Note: In hypertrophic cardiomyopathies, especially with outflow obstruction, an S_3 is common due to profound alteration in LV compliance.

THE PHYSIOLOGICAL VERSUS THE PATHOLOGICAL S_3

1. What is the difference in timing and quality between the physiological and the pathological S_3?

    ANS: None, except that the S_3 found in **constrictive pericarditis** may occur earlier than usual.

2. How can you usually tell a physiological from a pathological S_3?

    ANS: Only by knowing the circumstances under which it occurs, i.e., by finding the reason for the pathological S_3, such as symptoms and signs of heart failure or myocardial abnormalities.

    Note: Some patients with a pathological S_3 secondary to a past infarction are relatively asymptomatic, i.e., they do not seem to have the decreased exercise tolerance that is the usual consequence of a high left atrial V wave. The S_3 in these patients is often associated with a ventricular aneurysm or a large akinetic area. The mechanism for this S_3 is unknown.

3. Is the physiological S_3 ever as loud as the loudest pathological S_3?

    ANS: Almost. Conversely, a pathological S_3 may be very faint.

4. What noise may follow the pathological S_3? When is this heard with the physiological S_3?

    ANS: A short diastolic rumble is often heard following the pathological S_3. It is also heard with the torrential flow through the mitral valve that occurs when the physiological S_3 is exaggerated either by MR or by a PDA.

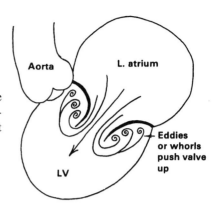

If the flow is fast, eddy currents may push the valve up enough to create a partial obstruction and so produce turbulent flow and a short diastolic murmur.

5. When does a high **filling pressure** not mean LV dysfunction and low ejection fraction?

ANS: If it is caused primarily by a high A wave, because a strong left atrial contraction can produce a high A wave at the end of diastole and so cause a high filling pressure, despite a normal ejection fraction. This is because it is the mean and not the end-diastolic filling pressure that best correlates with cardiac dysfunction. For example, in severe aortic stenosis there may be a 20-mm LV end-diastolic pressure but a mean left atrial pressure of 10 mm, and therefore no decreased function.

THE RIGHT VERSUS THE LEFT VENTRICULAR S$_3$

1. How can you tell whether an S$_3$ is from the RV or LV?

ANS: a. An S$_3$ generated by the RV is louder over the RV area, i.e., near the lower sternal area or epigastrium, unless the ventricle is markedly enlarged, in which case it may be loud over any part of the chest wall that overlies the RV. This includes those parts of the precordium usually occupied by the LV.

b. An RV S$_3$ is usually louder on inspiration because there is more flow into the RV. The LV S$_3$ may be louder on either inspiration or expiration. (See Question 2 under Loudness of the S$_3$ for explanation.)

c. An S$_3$ from the RV is usually associated with an RV heave or rock (see Chapter 5), a large jugular V wave, and a rapid Y descent.

2. List some of the common causes of an S$_3$ generated by the RV.

ANS: The common causes are RV dilatation and high right atrial pressures secondary to

a. Severe tricuspid regurgitation due to pulmonary hypertension.

b. Sudden RV outflow obstruction, as in massive pulmonary embolism.

THE S₃ VERSUS THE OPENING SNAP

1. What is the difference between the A_2–OS interval and the S_2–S_3 interval?

    ANS: The A_2–OS interval is rarely more than 100 ms (0.10 s), whereas the shortest A_2–S_3 interval is usually 120 ms (0.12 s). The difference between 100 and 120 ms is merely the difference between saying "pa-pa" as quickly as possible and saying it at a normal speaking rate.

2. How does the S_3 of a "tumor plop" differ from the usual S_3?

    ANS: A tumor plop is the early diastolic sound produced when a left (or right) atrial myxoma attached to a stalk prolapses through the mitral (or tricuspid) valve in diastole. This early diastolic sound can occur at the time one would expect either an OS or an S_3. It also differs from an S_3 by being more easily heard at the left lower sternal border than expected. (An S_3 is not usually heard at the left lower sternal border unless it is extremely loud.)

3. How does the site of best auscultation help to distinguish an S_3 from an OS?

    ANS: An OS is commonly loudest at some point between the apex and the left sternal border, whereas the S_3 is almost always loudest at the apex unless it is a right-sided S_3 or due to pericardial constriction.

    Note: In constrictive pericarditis, the early S_3 or pericardial knock, like the OS, may be loudest at the left sternal border, possibly because the RV also contributes to the early S_3 in this condition.

4. Why is the loud S_3 of pericardial constriction called a pericardial knock?

    ANS: Because it is very loud and there was controversy about calling it an S_3.

    Note: The pericardial knock is not present in **tamponade** because early rapid expansion of the ventricle is markedly blunted by the fluid.

Summary of How to Tell an S₃ from an Opening Snap

1. The OS is not usually more than 100 ms (a rapid "pa-pa") from the S_2. The S_3 is rarely less than 120 ms (0.12 s) from the A_2, i.e., a relaxed "two-three" interval.

2. The OS is usually a short, sharp click, best heard with the diaphragm near the left sternal border. The S_3 is a thud or boom, best heard by applying light or moderate pressure with the bell near the apex.

3. The OS is associated with a sharp, loud S_1. The S_3 may or may not have a loud S_1.

4. An OS will separate further from the A_2 when the patient stands. An S_3 will not change its distance from the A_2 on standing.

REFERENCES

1. Reddy, P. S., et al. The genesis of gallop sounds: Investigation by quantitative phono- and apexcardiography. *Circulation* 63:922,1981.
2. Schwartze, D. Frequency of the normal third heart sound in childhood. *Zeit. Kreislaufforschung* 55:306, 1966.
3. Wood, P The Eisenmenger syndrome or pulmonary hypertension with reversed central shunt. *Br. Med. J.* 2:701, 1958.

12 The Fourth Heart Sound (S₄)

NOMENCLATURE

1. What has the triple rhythm produced by the sequence of a fourth heart sound (S_4), the S_1, and the S_2 been called?

   ANS: An atrial gallop, a presystolic gallop, or an S_4 gallop.

   Note: a. The term *atrial gallop* implies that the atrium itself is the source of the extra sound. Atrial contraction itself is not audible with the stethoscope. It is the atrial effect on the ventricle that produces the sound. The atrium and ventricle are analogous to a drumstick and drum. The drumstick (atrium) is necessary in order to produce the sound, but the drum (ventricle) actually generates the sound.

   b. The term *presystolic gallop* is misleading because the gallop sound produced by an S_3 may also be "presystolic" during a tachycardia, when the first sound follows very shortly after the S_3.

2. What is the advantage of the term S_4?

   ANS: It specifies exactly which extra sound is thought to be producing the triple rhythm, regardless of diastolic length and without reference to exact mechanisms. It enables you to refer to the single sound S_4 without the necessity of always using the term *gallop*, which by definition implies at least three sounds.

MODE OF PRODUCTION

1. Where is the S_4 best recorded by an intracardiac phonocatheter, in the atrium or in the ventricle?

   ANS: In the ventricle.

2. What does the apex cardiogram (apex impulse tracing) show at the time of the S_4?

   ANS: It shows a hump just before the systolic outward impulse. This presystolic hump or A wave is often large enough to be palpable.

   Note: The peak of the A wave coincides with the largest vibration of the S_4.

3. What causes this A wave or end-diastolic outward movement on the apex cardiogram?

> ANS: It is the effect of left atrial contraction, causing a slight increase in the volume of the left ventricle (LV) at the end of diastole. This slight increase in volume before the ventricle contracts can be seen even in normal subjects on a cineangiogram with contrast material in the LV.

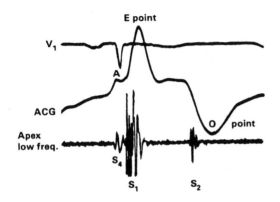

Apex cardiogram and phonocardiogram from a 50-year-old man with a previous infarction. The S_4 is simultaneous with a large palpable atrial hump (A wave) on the apex cardiogram. The A wave is 15% of the total apex pulse amplitude, or vertical E to O distance. Atrial humps of 15% or more of the E–O amplitude are usually palpable.

> *Note*: An apical A wave may be palpable even when the S_4 may be too low in frequency to be audible. On the other hand, a pathological S_4 may be heard in the absence of a palpable A wave. This is obvious when you realize that only a chest that allows an apex beat to be easily palpated will allow you to palpate the A wave, yet the S_4 sound may still be heard.

4. Can an S_4 be produced by an atrium that is contracting against a stenotic atrioventricular (AV) valve as in mitral stenosis (MS)?

> ANS: No. The atrium must be able to transmit its pressure freely to the LV, or else only a presystolic murmur will be heard.

5. What theory could account for the production of an audible S_4 if it (a) occurs at the peak of atrial contraction, (b) causes such an increase in LV end-diastolic volume that it produces a recordable and often palpable systolic outward movement, and (c) is recorded best in the ventricle?

> ANS: Atrial contraction, by causing eddy currents on the undersurface of the AV valves, tends to hold them upward. However, since atrial contraction also raises the volume in the ventricle, the chordae tendineae and papillary muscles are stretched at exactly the same time as the AV valves are being pulled up or held in the opposite direction. If it has enough energy, this tug on the chordae and papillary muscles could account for the sound.

RECOGNIZING THE RHYTHM OF THE S₄ GALLOP

If you remember that the P wave indirectly produces the S_4 and the QRS is indirectly responsible for the S_1, then, if you know that the S_2 occurs at the end of the T, the rhythm of S_4, S_1, and S_2 is the same as that of P, QRS, and the end of T.

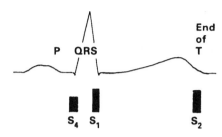

If you realize that the T wave is a systolic event, it will be easy to remember that the S_2 comes at the end of the T wave. Thus, the rhythm of an S_4 gallop is the rhythm symbolized by PR—T, where R represents the QRS complex and T represents the end of the T.

Because the P is closer to the QRS than the QRS is to the end of the T, the rhythm or cadence of an S_4 gallop is a pair of sounds close together followed by a pause, then the second sound. Therefore, the rhythm of two cycles would be as follows 4-1——2——4-1——2.

Vocal imitations of the heart sounds can help in perceiving the actual phenomena. Because the S_4 is low-pitched, you should practice imitating the S_4-S_1——S_2 by saying "huh-one——two." Place the "huh" as closely as possible to the "one," so that they are practically one word: "huh-one." Also, say the "huh" as softly as possible, because the S_4 is often just within the realm of audibility. Like the S_3, it is also volume- and proximity-dependent so that it tends to range in and out of audibility from beat to beat when it is soft.

THE PHYSIOLOGICAL S₄

1. Can an S_4 be heard in normal subjects?

    ANS: It can occasionally be heard in some normal subjects in all age groups. However, it is so rarely normal that unless it is heard in an athlete or a subject whose daily work is physical and who has physiological hypertrophy, you should suspect that it is an abnormal finding.

    Note: About 50% of athletes (e.g., professional basketball players) have a physiological S_4 [1].

THE PATHOLOGICAL S₄

Causes and Associated Conditions

1. When should you consider an S_4 pathological?

    ANS: You should consider any S_4 possibly pathological, even in a young subject, until proved otherwise. This means that before you call it physiological in the younger age group, you should probably hear a physiological S_3 and a physiologically split S_2, feel a normal apex beat, hear a venous hum in the neck (see Chapter 14), and obtain a normal ECG, chest X-ray, and echocardiogram to rule out a hypertrophic cardiomyopathy.

2. What condition generates a strong enough atrial contraction to produce an audible S_4?

    ANS: Any condition in which the ventricle is "stiffer" than normal, i.e., in which the ventricle has decreased distensibility or **compliance**.

3. How does loss of distensibility of a ventricle cause a strong atrial contraction, i.e., how does the atrium "know" it must contract more strongly when the ventricle has lost compliance?

    ANS: While the mitral valve is open, pressures are almost equal in both atrium and ventricle. This common diastolic chamber may be called an atrioventricle. If the LV is poorly distensible, as with left ventricular hypertrophy (LVH), the pressure rise due to filling of the atrioventricle from the pulmonary veins is steep. By the time the P wave and its subsequent atrial contraction occur, the atrial pressure is so high that, via a strong Starling effect, the atrium will contract with greater energy than normal.

4. What conditions cause a decreased compliance of the ventricle?

    ANS: Those in which the ventricle is

    a. Thickened by LVH, as when it is laboring under a chronic pressure load, e g, hypertension (the most common cause of LVH in which an S_4 is heard) and in hypertrophic **cardiomyopathies**.

    b. Stiffened by replacement of myocardium by fibrous tissue, e.g., an old myocardial infarction.

    c. Stiffened by ischemia due to angina or acute infarction. (Subtotal or total acute coronary occlusions in dogs increases the stiffness of the LV [2].)

    Note: A patient whose filling pressure is elevated by a strong atrial contraction will be less dyspneic than one who has the same high filling pressure due to a high V wave, because a high A wave starting from a low

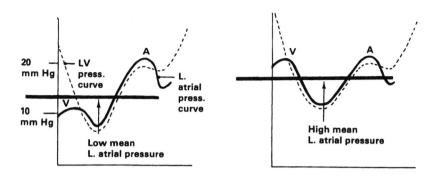

A low V wave and a disproportionately high A wave are seen on the left. These give a lower mean left atrial pressure and therefore less dyspnea than do both a high V wave and a relatively poor atrial contraction, as seen on the right.

left atrial pressure will result in a lower mean left atrial pressure than will a high V wave falling to a high left atrial pressure.

5. What causes an atrium in sinus rhythm to be too weak to help out a ventricle?

   ANS: a. Atrial damage.

             b. Too little blood in the atrium, e.g., due to diuresis.

             c. The influence of agents that decrease inotropism, such as beta blockers.

6. How can the S₄ assist in the diagnosis of **constrictive pericarditis** or **tamponade**? Explain.

   ANS: An S₄ is not heard in constriction or tamponade. This is because:

             a. The ventricle is unable to expand at the end of diastole due to the constriction.

             b. The atrium may be so tethered by the constrictive process that it cannot contract well.

The S₄ in Myocardial Infarction

1. What proportion of patients with acute myocardial infarction have an S₄?

   ANS: Almost all will have a phonocardiographic S₄ unless they have MS or atrial infarction. It is heard by auscultation in about half of the patients during the first few days following infarction [2].

   Note: An infarcted area, whether dyskinetic (bulges out like an **aneurysm** in systole) or akinetic (no movement during systole), causes loss of compliance of the LV. Presence of excess catecholamines, which is usual in the first few days of infarction, can also cause a loss of compliance of the LV [3].

The S_4 in Volume Overloads

1. When is ventricular enlargement usually associated with a normally compliant ventricle, and therefore with an absent S_4?

    ANS: When the volume overload is chronic due to regurgitation or shunt flows, i.e., in **ventricular septal defect** (VSD), **persistent ductus arteriosus** (PDA), chronic aortic regurgitation (AR), or chronic mitral regurgitation (MR).

2. When will there be an S_4 in a subject with MR?

    ANS: When the MR is

    a. Secondary to papillary muscle dysfunction or LV dilatation due to fibrosis or ischemia.

    b. Sudden and severe due to ruptured chordae. In this cause, the left atrium and ventricle are enlarged only moderately despite the massive volume overload, probably because the pericardium resists acute stretching.

    Note: In rheumatic, chronic MR, there is almost never a left-sided S_4 partly because the left atrium is dilated, damaged, and hypocontractile.

LOUDNESS AND AUDIBILITY OF THE S_4 ─────────────

1. Where is the LV S_4 usually best heard?

    ANS: At the apex, when the patient is in the left lateral decubitus position.

2. Why should you usually use the stethoscope bell to bring out the S_4?

    ANS: An S_3 or an S_4 may occasionally be heard better with firm bell pressure, which reduces the volume inside the bell. It may be that the volume displacement by the A wave into a smaller total volume produces a greater effect on the eardrum.

3. Why is held expiration as a means of bringing the stethoscope closer to the heart a poor method of bringing out a soft S_4?

    ANS: Held respiration (apnea) will decrease venous return because the lungs act like a pump and help speed up the circulation time. This soft S_4 is very sensitive to blood volume.

4. How can the S_4 be made louder besides increasing blood flow to the atrium?

    ANS: a. By bringing ventricular movements closer to the stethoscope.
    b. Handgrip.

5. Besides having the patient exercise, how can you increase the flow to the atrium?

    ANS: a. By asking the patient to release a Valsalva strain that has been maintained for at least 10 s. This will cause a sudden rush of blood to the right ventricle (RV) and a few seconds later to the LV, which then also must pump against an increased resistance for several seconds after the Valsalva strain.

b. By asking the patient to cough several times. This is really another form of exercise as well as a mini-Valsalva maneuver.

c. By asking the patient to take four or five deep, rapid breaths. This activates the lung pump and thus increases flow to the heart.

d. By asking the patient to squat. This can increase the cardiac output for a few beats.

e. By isometric contraction through a handgrip (see below for hemodynamics). This increases cardiac output as well as blood pressure.

6. How can you bring ventricular movement closer to the stethoscope?

   ANS: Turn the patient to the left lateral decubitus position. (If you listen immediately afterward, the effect of the exertion will also be operative for a few beats.)

   Note: When all these maneuvers fail to produce an S_4 that is suspected, have the patient change from a standing to a left lateral decubitus position. This often produces an S_4 for a few beats.

7. When does isometric handgrip contraction, such as when one squeezes a folded towel with one hand, bring out an S_4?

   ANS: When there is decreased LV function.

8. How does handgrip contraction increase blood pressure?

   ANS: Handgrip produces local ischemia, which generates reflexes whose apparent purpose is to supply more blood flow to the ischemic area. Handgrip transiently increases cardiac output through an augmentation of heart rate and contractility. It also increases peripheral resistance in hypertensive patients and in patients with a reduction in cardiac reserve [4].

DIFFERENTIATION OF THE S₄ FROM THE S₃

1. How does the quality or pitch of the S_4 differ from that of the S_3?

   ANS: They do not differ. They may both be described as a low-pitched thud or boom.

   Note: Because of their very low frequency of vibrations, they often feel more like a physical "pop" or movement felt by the eardrum than like a sound.

2. How can you tell without a phonocardiogram or pulse tracing whether an S_3 or an S_4 is present when a tachycardia causes confusion?

   ANS: a. If you can slow the rate with carotid sinus pressure, you may be able to discern that the extra sound keeps a constant relationship to the S_1, in which case it is an S_4. If it maintains a constant relationship to the S_2 and moves away from the S_1, it is an S_3.

b. Wait for a pause following a premature beat. An S_4 precedes the S_1 that ends the pause.

3. If both an S_3 and an S_4 are present, what is the rhythm called?

ANS: Quadruple rhythm, train-wheel rhythm, or double gallop.

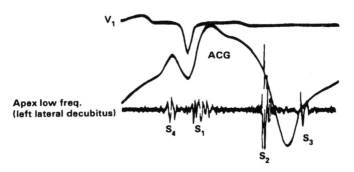

Apex impulse tracing (apex cardiogram) from a 55-year-old man with two previous infarctions. Surprisingly, despite his double gallop, he was almost asymptomatic without treatment.

DIFFERENTIATION OF AN S_4–S_1 FROM A SPLIT S_1 (M_1–A_1 or M_1–T_1)

1. What is the difference in quality between an S_4 and the first major component of a split S_1, i.e., the M_1?

ANS: When the S_4 is loud, it is difficult to tell the difference in quality between an S_4 and an M_1, but when soft, the S_4 has fewer high frequencies, so that it is often inaudible when the diaphragm is pressed hard against the chest. The M_1 is usually heard almost as well with the diaphragm as with the bell, regardless of whether it is loud or soft.

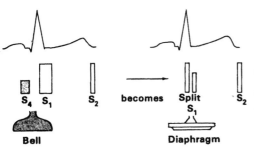

The use of a diaphragm will eliminate most soft S_4s and may bring out the narrow, sharp, clicking physiological split of S_1.

2. How can the site of auscultation tell you whether you are listening to an S_4–S_1 rather than to a split M_1–A_1 or M_1–T_1?

     ANS: The S_4 is very sensitive to proximity and tends to disappear anywhere away from the apex beat. Therefore, a split S_1 that sounds the same at the left sternal border as at the apex has an M_1 as the first component.

3. How can postural volume changes differentiate an S_4 from an M_1–A_1?

     ANS: Because the S_4 is very sensitive to blood volume changes, standing will generally make it disappear. The M_1–A_1 may even become more apparent on standing because the M_1–A_1 interval represents isovolumic contraction time, which can be prolonged by standing, and wide splits are more obvious to the ear.

     Note: A general principle to help you distinguish an S_4 from an M_1 is that it is easy to get rid of an S_4. If the first component of what sounds like a split S_1 disappears on decreasing blood volumes, on increasing stethoscope pressure, or by moving away from the apex, you are dealing with an S_4. If the S_4 is so loud that none of the above maneuvers diminish it, it will usually be palpable as an atrial hump or A wave on the apex beat's pulse contour with the patient in the left lateral decubitus position.

SEVERITY OF CARDIAC DYSFUNCTION AND PRESENCE OF AN S₄

1. What does the presence of an S_4 indicate about the gradient in (a) aortic stenosis (AS) and (b) pulmonary stenosis (PS)?

     ANS: a. In valvular AS it suggests a severe gradient of at least 70 mmHg across the aortic valve [5]. This is not valid either in subjects with angina, in whom ischemic heart disease may be an additional cause of an S_4, or in subjects with hypertrophic obstructive cardiomyopathy (HOCM), who may have an S_4 with any gradient.

         b. In PS it also suggests a gradient across the pulmonary valve or infundibulum of at least 70 mmHg.

2. Which is a more serious sign of heart disease, the pathological left-sided S_3 or the S_4?

     ANS: A pathological S_3 is more serious because it is associated with both a stiff ventricle and an increase in left atrial V-wave pressure. The latter is a sign of decompensation at rest. An S_4, on the other hand, merely means that there is only a poorly compliant ventricle which is "calling on the atrium for help," i.e., there is only a high A-wave pressure. The help that the ventricle receives may be enough to keep the output adequate even with moderate exercise.

Note: An S_4 tends to rule out restrictive or constrictive myocardial disease, e.g., amyloid, tamponade, or constrictive pericarditis.

THE S_4–S_1 INTERVAL AND SEVERITY OF DYSFUNCTION ————

1. What is the relationship between the S_4–S_1 interval and the severity of the loss of compliance present?

    ANS: The shorter the P–S_4 interval the more severe is the loss of compliance [6]. This means that the longer the S_4–S_1 interval, the more severe is the loss of compliance.

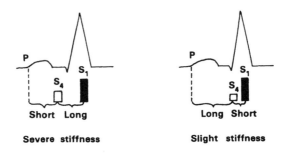

The longer the S_4–S_1 interval, the greater is the loss of compliance of the LV (provided the P–R interval is not prolonged) and usually the louder is the S_4.

2. How does the S_4–S_1 interval affect S_4 and S_1 loudness?

    ANS: a. The earlier the S_4, the louder it becomes.

    Note: By electrical pacing of dogs' atria it has been shown that the earlier in diastole the atrium contracts, the more powerfully it contracts, so long S_4–S_1 intervals result in a more energetic ventricular contraction than do short S_4–S_1 intervals.

    b. As the S_4 moves farther from the S_1, the S_1 becomes softer.

SUMMATION AND AUGMENTED GALLOPS ————

1. Why can a first-degree AV block augment the S_4?

    ANS: A first-degree AV block, i.e., in which the P waves come relatively early in diastole, may cause the atrium to contract early enough to coincide with rapid ventricular filling. Atrial contraction occurring at this time squeezes blood into the ventricle at the same time that rapid ventricular expansion is also drawing blood into the ventricle. Thus, a soft S_4 can become very loud. Unless the P–R interval is extremely prolonged, this contraction of the atrium at the time of rapid ventricular filling will occur only with a tachycardia.

2. What is the gallop rhythm called when the high flow of the early rapid filling phase of the LV is augmented by atrial contraction, as with first-degree AV block and tachycardia?

   ANS: A summation gallop, i.e., it is the summation of the mechanism for the production of an S_3 with the mechanism for the production of an S_4, to make an audible sound.

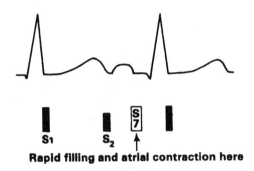

Rapid filling and atrial contraction here

Simultaneous occurrence of atrial contraction and early rapid filling produces a summation sound facetiously called the "S7" ($S_3 + S_4$). This usually requires a prolonged P–R interval.

Note: A summation gallop is physiological if neither an S_3 nor an S_4 would be present without the first-degree AV block and tachycardia.

3. When are summation gallops pathological?

   ANS: When a pathological S_3 is augmented by atrial contraction occurring very early in diastole or when a pathological S_4 is augmented by occurring during the rapid filling phase. These are then called "augmented gallops." This implies that a pathological S_3 or an S_4 was augmented by the fortuitous assistance of a marked tachycardia or prolonged P–R interval.

   Note: a. Summation sounds are very loud even if not pathological.
   b. If the heart rate of a patient with a physiological summation gallop is slowed by carotid sinus pressure, you may hear nothing but an S_1 and S_2. (The carotid sinus is level with the upper border of the thyroid cartilage.)

   c. The summation gallop often has some duration and can mimic a mid-diastolic murmur.

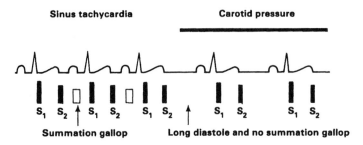

Carotid pressure slows the heart rate and separates the time of atrial contraction from the time of early rapid ventricular filling, thus eliminating a summation gallop.

THE PACEMAKER S_4-LIKE CLICK

1. When can an electronic pacemaker produce an extra sound? When does the extra sound occur?

   ANS: When it causes intercostal skeletal muscle contraction, it can produce a high-pitched, clicking sound just preceding the M_1, so that it sounds like a widely split S_1. It is accentuated by inspiration and occurs about 6 ms after the pacing stimulus. Perforation of the myocardium of the RV by a transvenous pacing electrode should be suspected when the pacemaker-induced sound occurs. This, however, is not a necessary concomitant.

REFERENCES

1. Roeske, W. R., et al. Noninvasive study of athletes' hearts. *Circulation* 53:287,1976.
2. Stock, E. Auscultation and phonocardiography in acute myocardial infarction. *Med. J. Austral.* 1:1060, 1966.
3. Diamond, G., and Forrester, J. S. Effects of coronary artery disease and acute myocardial infarction on left ventricular compliance in man. *Circulation* 45:11, 1972.
4. Matthews, O. A., et al. Left ventricular function during isometric exercise (handgrip): Significance of an atrial gallop (S_4). *Am. Heart J.* 88:686, 1974.
5. Goldblatt, A., Aygen, M. D., and Braunwald, E. Hemodynamic phonocardiographic correlations of the fourth heart sound in aortic stenosis. *Circulation* 26:92, 1962.
6. Duchosal, P. A study of gallop rhythm by a combination of phonocardiographic and electrocardiographic methods. *Am. Heart J.* 7:613, 1932.

13 Ejection Murmurs

PHYSICAL CAUSES

1. What is the cause of murmurs?

    ANS: Sufficient flow in the cardiovascular system to generate enough tur-
    bulent energy in the walls of the heart or blood vessels to produce
    sounds. High-energy turbulence can be produced by either obstruc-
    tion to blood flow or flow into a distal chamber of larger diameter
    than the proximal one.

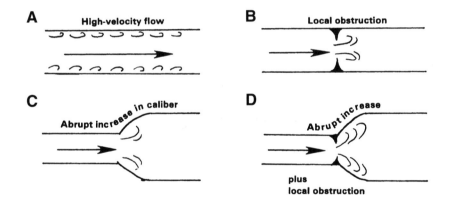

Causes of turbulence. In **A**, turbulence occurs in fluids flowing at high velocity
through tubes of uniform caliber, according to the formula for Reynolds numbers.
In **B** and **C**, either a local obstruction or fluid flowing into a channel of larger diameter can produce turbulence at much less flow velocity. In **D**, a combined effect of
obstruction and abrupt increase in caliber, as in poststenotic dilatation, produces
turbulence at relatively low flow velocity.

2. What happens to the velocity of flow at an orifice?

    ANS: It increases, just as it does when you narrow the nozzle of a hose.

3. How does a decrease in orifice area affect the volume of flow across it, the rate of flow across it, and the loudness of the murmur?

   ANS: With a decrease in orifice area, the volume of flow will tend to be maintained by a compensatory increase in pressure upstream from the stenotic area. The smaller the orifice, the greater is the velocity of flow at the orifice and the greater the turbulence and the loudness of the murmur.

   Note: Turbulence is also affected by the following factors:

   a. Viscosity. The greater the viscosity, the less is the turbulence. It is to be expected, then, that the high hematocrit in patients with cyanotic congenital heart disease can increase blood viscosity enough to attenuate murmurs.

   b. The irregularity and sharpness of the edge of the orifice. The greater the irregularity or sharpness at the orifice edges, the louder the murmur. This may account for the surprisingly loud ejection murmurs in some elderly patients with aortic valve sclerosis.

4. How does the frequency or pitch of a murmur relate to the (a) **gradient** and (b) flow?

   ANS: a. The greater the gradient, the higher are the frequency and pitch produced. High gradients with little flow volume produce "blowing murmurs."

   b. The greater the flow, the more low and medium frequencies are produced ("the greater the flow, the more the low"). When low gradients produce murmurs that are highly dependent on flow, the result is a "rumbling murmur," e.g., mitral stenosis diastolic murmurs.

   c. A combination of high gradient and high flow produces mixed frequencies which, if loud, can result in harsh murmurs.

CHARACTERISTICS OF THE EJECTION MURMUR _____

1. What valvular flow event is implied by the term *ejection murmur*?

   ANS: The term implies a murmur that is produced by blood flowing forward through a semilunar valve (aortic or pulmonary valve) during systole.

2. What is characteristic of ejection murmurs on a phonocardiogram?

   ANS: They start with the final component of the first heart sound (S_1); are diamond, rhomboid, or kite-shaped; and finish before the second sound of the side of the heart from which the murmur originates. This means that a left-sided ejection murmur will finish before the A_2, and a right-sided ejection murmur will finish before the P_2.

Boldface type indicates that the term is explained in the glossary.

3. Why must an ejection murmur be crescendo–decrescendo in loudness?

   ANS: The configuration and loudness of a murmur across a valve is controlled mainly by the shape of the gradient. This gradient is proportional to the velocity and acceleration of flow.

   In aortic stenosis (AS), as the pressure in the left ventricle (LV) rises to just above diastolic pressure in the aorta, it takes a short time to overcome the inertia of the aortic blood and walls. Therefore, the initial gradient across the aortic orifice is slight, and the murmur starts softly.

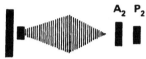 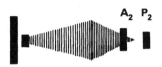

This murmur could be either pulmonary or aortic, since it ends before both components of the second sound.

This murmur may be a pulmonary ejection murmur, since, although it extends beyond the A_2, it finishes before the P_2.

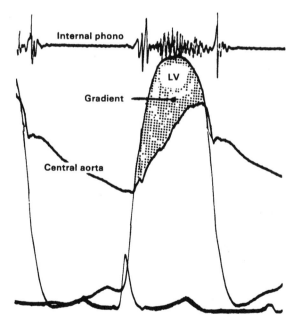

A simultaneous aortic and LV pressure tracing (taken with a catheter-tip micromanometer to eliminate time delays through tubes) in a subject with valvular AS. The shape of the murmur follows the shape of the gradient (shaded area).

The pressure gradient and velocity of flow then increases toward mid-systole, as does the murmur. As soon as the ventricle begins to reach the stage of reduced ejection, just past the middle of systole, the flow decreases, and the murmur decreases.

Just before the valve closes, the velocity of forward flow has decreased so much that even if the murmur does extend to the second sound by phonocardiogram, the ear cannot hear the very end of this faint decrescendo part of the murmur.

The decrescendo at the end of an ejection murmur is steep enough so that if the murmur is short, with the peak early in systole, a pause before the S_2 is easily perceived. Such a murmur and obvious pause suggests a small gradient. (See figure on p. 198.) However, if the stenosis is more than mild, the peak may reach mid-systole with no obvious pause between the end of the murmur and the S_2, and it may be difficult to know that it is not a pansystolic regurgitant murmur. However, if the ejection murmur is louder than the S_2, the steep decrescendo allows you to hear even a very soft S_2. A regurgitant murmur that is louder than the S_2 will eliminate any S_2 that is not louder than the murmur.

4. What happens to the loudness of an ejection murmur after a long diastole, as in the long pause after a premature ventricular contraction or after the long diastoles of atrial fibrillation? Why?

   ANS: It becomes louder because

   a. The long period of diastole allows a larger volume to collect in the LV and stretch its walls. This increased volume is ejected during the next systole with increased energy by means of the Starling effect.
   b. A long diastole allows more peripheral runoff and therefore a reduction in afterload. This causes an increase in the velocity of myocardial shortening and an increase in the volume of forward flow.
   c. The **postextrasystolic potentiation** following an early ventricular depolarization (as with premature ectopic beats) produces a positive inotropic effect on the ventricle and contributes to the loudness of the ejection.

5. Why do the pitch or frequency characteristics of an ejection murmur not change when the murmur is soft?

   ANS: Ejection murmurs are produced by the entire stroke volume passing through the aortic or pulmonary valves with each systole. Therefore there will always be enough flow to produce low and medium frequencies, even when the obstruction or gradient across the valve is trivial. This is not true for regurgitant murmurs.

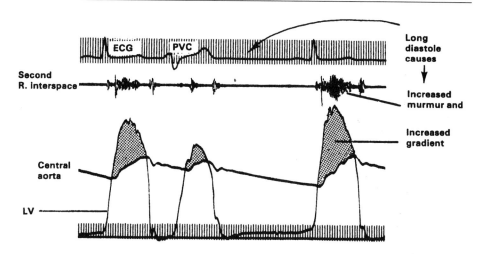

A phonocardiogram and simultaneous aortic and LV pressure tracing from a 16-year-old boy with valvular AS. Not only did the murmur and gradient increase after the long diastole, but the ejection sound also increased. Note that the small gradient of the premature ventricular contraction (PVC) itself produced only a short early systolic murmur.

6. How can you best define an ejection murmur?

   ANS: It is best defined as an "ejection murmur complex," i.e., it is a murmur that begins at the end of the S_1, is crescendo–decrescendo, ends before the second sound of its side, becomes louder after long diastoles, and retains low and medium frequencies even when soft.

7. How can you tell by auscultation that a murmur is markedly crescendo–decrescendo?

   ANS: A rhythmic cadence is created by the sequence of the S_1 followed by the peak of the crescendo followed by the S_2:

huh–huh–duh

S_1 Peak S_2
of
diamond

   Note: If an S_2 is missing, the rhythm of "huh–huh" tells you that the murmur is crescendo–decrescendo. If the S_1 is missing, the rhythm of "huh–duh" also tells you that the murmur is crescendo–decrescendo.

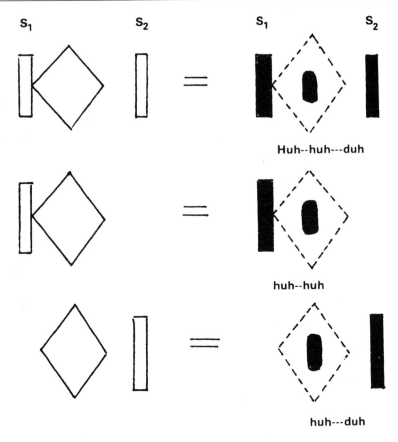

The peak of the ejection murmur produces a recognizable cadence or rhythm even if only one of the heart sounds is present.

8. How can the loudness of an ejection murmur tell you whether or not there is a significant gradient across a valve?

   ANS: A soft murmur, i.e., grade 2 or less, is likely to signify an unimportant gradient, provided that artifactual reasons for the softness, such as obesity or heart failure, are absent. If the murmur is very loud, i.e., grade 4/6 or more, the gradient is likely to be at least 20 mmHg. Unfortunately, a loud murmur does not tell you how much over 20 mmHg the gradient may be.

9. List some factors, besides a thin chest wall, that spuriously increase the loudness of systolic ejection murmurs, i.e., without reflecting the degree of the gradient.

   ANS: Any cause of increased flow, such as exercise, thyrotoxicosis, arteriovenous fistula, anemia, shunt, or excessive diastolic filling, as in bradycardia or aortic regurgitation.

TYPES OF EJECTION MURMURS

1. List the two common types of ejection murmurs.

    ANS: a. The systolic flow murmur, i.e., a murmur due to causes other than obstruction to flow.
    b. The aortic or pulmonary stenosis ejection murmur.

2. List the five types of systolic flow murmurs.

    ANS: a. The murmur due to the normal "impulse gradient," which is perceivable only because of a thin chest or quiet room. A normal impulse gradient is the gradient produced by the normal acceleration of ventricular blood across a nonobstructed semilunar valve.
    b. The flow murmur due to increased stroke volume or rate of ejection.
    c. The murmur due to unknown anatomical causes of turbulence, namely the innocent humming ejection murmur of childhood.
    d. The murmur due to aortic sclerosis.
    e. The murmur due to ejection into a dilated artery.

    Note: The three major examples of this latter type of murmur are idiopathic dilatation of the pulmonary artery or of the ascending aorta, as with an **aneurysm**, and the pulmonary ejection murmur occurring in patients with severe pulmonary hypertension. These murmurs are very short, finishing at about mid-systole.

SYSTOLIC FLOW MURMURS

The Normal Impulse Gradient Murmur and the Increased Flow Murmur

1. How can a systolic murmur be produced across a normal semilunar valve?

    ANS: There is always a forward pressure gradient across a semilunar valve, as there must be in any pipe with a forward flow.

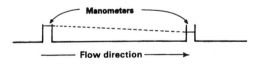

The gradient between the upstream and downstream manometers may not be measurable by the usual cardiac catheter techniques. If, however, the gradient is increased enough by obstruction to flow, a semilunar valve, or even a local protuberance from one wall, enough turbulence may occur to produce a murmur.

2. What is the relationship between the gradient across the semilunar valve and the shape of the murmur?

>   ANS: The greater the gradient across a semilunar valve, the louder and longer the murmur and the later the peak of the crescendo–decrescendo.

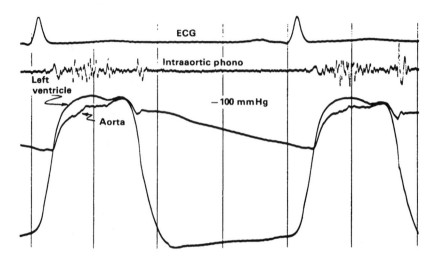

>   Aortic and LV pressure tracings together with a phonocardiogram from a 40-year-old man with an innocent aortic ejection murmur. Note the early systolic gradient between the LV and aorta, which is the normal impulse gradient found not only in normal left-sided chambers but also normally seen between the right ventricle and pulmonary artery. This tracing is taken by a single catheter with two end holes, in order to obtain absolutely accurate timing and pressure differences across the aortic valve.

3. In what percentage of normal subjects is the normal impulse gradient ejection murmur heard?

>   ANS: In 100%, depending on
>
>   >   a. The soundproofing of the room. All normal subjects have an ejection murmur in a soundproof room, usually along the left sternal border [1].
>   >   b. The age of the subject. About 90% of healthy children up to age 14 have ejection murmurs on ordinary clinical examination in a quiet but not soundproof room [2]. 'These murmurs are usually maximal at the left sternal border. About 15% of adults under age 40 have an innocent ejection murmur.

Ejection Murmurs Due to Increased Flow

1. What are the preferred terms for an easily audible ejection murmur that is produced by an increase in flow across a valve rather than by a valve narrowing?

   ANS: a. *Systolic flow murmur* is the preferred term when speaking to physicians.

   b. *Innocent murmur* is the preferred term when speaking to patients. This term implies that the prognosis is such that it will give the patient no trouble. This is a very reassuring term to use in speaking to a patient.

   Note: "Benign" and "functional" are not desirable terms. Benign implies that an abnormality is present but is not malignant. Functional may have no meaning to a layperson, although to a physician it may mean "due to increased flow."

2. List the most common causes of ejection flow murmurs due to increased stroke volume.

   ANS: a. Shunt flow, e.g., due to an **atrial septal defect** (ASD) or **ventricular septal defect** (VSD).

   b. Increased ventricular volumes caused by
   (1) Regurgitant leaks such as aortic or pulmonary regurgitation.
   (2) Pregnancy.
   (3) Marked bradycardia, as in complete **atrioventricular block**.

   c. Increased cardiac output, as in thyrotoxicosis, anemia, exercise, and systemic arteriovenous fistulas.

   Note: Cardiac output is not significantly increased in anemia until the hemoglobin and hematocrit drop to about 50 percent of normal. Patients with anemia may have a lower viscosity than normal, and this may also increase turbulence.

3. What is meant by a "hemic" murmur?

   ANS: A hemic murmur is any murmur that is present in the anemic state and disappears when the anemia is corrected. For example, mitral regurgitation (MR) may be heard only with the increased heart size, blood volume, and need for coronary flow caused by severe anemia [3].

Atrial Septal Defect Systolic Flow Murmurs

1. What causes a systolic murmur in patients with an uncomplicated ASD?

   ANS: Increased flow through the dilated main pulmonary artery.

2. Why is there no murmur through the defect in the atrial septum?

    ANS: Because there is almost no gradient across the defect. If the defect is large, the two atria act as a single chamber, so that the pressures on each side of the defect are almost equal. Even if the defect is small, the gradient between the left and right atria is never more than a few millimeters of mercury.

3. Where is the ASD systolic ejection murmur best heard?

    ANS: At the second or third left interspace.

    Note: The marked increase in pulmonary flow may generate systolic flow murmurs, best heard over the upper back or in the axilla. They may increase with inspiration.

4. What suggests that part of the pulmonary flow murmur of ASD is often extracardiac, i.e., probably due to adhesions between the dilated pulmonary artery and the pleura?

    ANS: a. It is often crackly, crunchy, or scratchy.
          b. Other causes of marked pulmonary artery dilatation sometimes produce this crackling or crunchy type of murmur (e.g., idiopathic dilatation of the pulmonary artery).
          c. It is often louder and longer than a mere flow murmur should be despite the absence of pulmonary stenosis (PS).
          d. In some ASDs there is no ejection murmur, despite at least a moderate silent.

5. What condition can mimic the murmur and S_2 of an ASD?

    ANS: Idiopathic dilatation of the pulmonary artery: they both can have crunchy murmurs and a delayed P_2.

The Straight Back Syndrome Ejection Murmur

1. What is meant by the straight back syndrome?

    ANS: Compression of the heart due to loss of the normal dorsal curvature of the spine, resulting in a pulmonary ejection murmur that is usually mistaken for that of either PS or ASD.

2. Why will loss of the normally gentle dorsal kyphosis cause a pulmonary ejection murmur?

    ANS: The upper mediastinal structures, including the pulmonary artery, may be compressed against the sternum, and can actually produce a gradient of 5–15 mmHg across the pulmonary outflow tract.

Note: An anteroposterior chest diameter (back of sternum to front of vertebrae) that is one-third or less of the transverse diameter (from the inside
of the ribs), measured at just above the right dome of the diaphragm, is
almost diagnostic of the straight back syndrome.

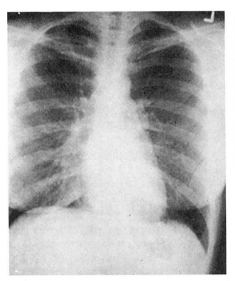 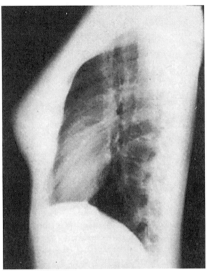

If this patient with a loss of dorsal curvature, the anteroposterior diameter of the internal aspect of the chest (from back of sternum to front of vertebrae) is one-third of the
transverse diameter. (Courtesy of Dr. Antonio C. deLeon, Jr.).

The Humming Systolic Ejection Murmur

1. What adjectives have been used to describe the quality, or timber, of the humming (innocent) ejection murmur that is found in children? What eponym has
   been used for it?

   ANS: It has been described as a buzzing, vibratory, twanging, moaning, or
   groaning murmur. It has also been called *Still's murmur*, after the Brit-
   ish author of a pediatric textbook published in 1918, who described it
   as a "twanging string" murmur.

2. Why was it thought by some to be an aortic murmur?

   ANS: A fine vibration can sometimes be recorded on the carotid tracing, and
   the aortic root is thought by some to be relatively narrow in some of
   these patients.

3. What does the humming or vibratory quality of the murmur tell you about the prognosis?

   ANS: It strongly suggests that the murmur is innocent and will probably (but not always) disappear after puberty.

4. Where is the humming murmur usually heard best?

   ANS: Although it is best heard between the apex and the left sternal border, it is surprising how widespread it is and how difficult it is to localize it.

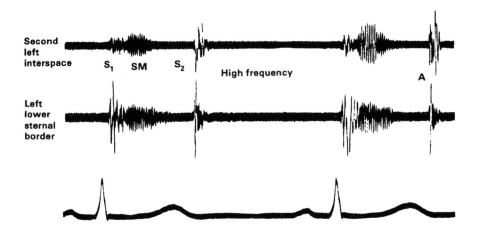

The regular vibrations on this phonocardiogram of a humming systolic murmur (SM) tell you that the murmur has a musical quality. The peak of the crescendo occurring in the first third of systole tells you that the gradient across the semilunar valve is probably trivial.

5. What suggests that it is a form of "flow" ejection murmur and is not due to obstruction?

   ANS: a. The murmur is never louder than grade 3/6, and often disappears when the subject stands.
   b. The murmur is usually short and reaches its peak early.
   c. It is often associated with a venous hum (see Chapter 14).
   d. It consists mostly of low and medium frequencies, i.e., between 75 and 160 cps. A murmur that is relatively low in pitch suggests that it is due mostly to flow with very little gradient.

   Note: These humming murmurs may become as long as important murmurs in the presence of further increases blood flow, such as that occurring with high fever or severe anemia.

6. What suggests that this murmur may actually be a "twanging string" murmur as originally described by Still.

> ANS: Most children with this murmur have a threadlike false tendon, over 60% of which stretches across the outflow tract of the left ventricle.

The Aortic Sclerosis Murmur

1. What percentage of patients over age 50 have an easily audible aortic ejection murmur without valvular stenosis?

> ANS: About 50%. Echoardioqrams have shown that many elderly patients have a septum that bends into the outflow tract, the so-called sigmoid septum (sigma = Greek S). This could create enough turbulence to mimic the murmur of aortic valve sclerosis (sclerosis = Greek "hard"). Therefore a more nonspecific terminology should be used. Since about 50% of patients over age 50 have the murmur especially if they are hypertensive, we should call this the "50 over 50" (50/50) murmur. However, if you eliminate patients with elevated blood pressure and ECG evidence of LVH, then only about 30% will have this murmur [4].

2. What are the causes of an innocent aortic ejection murmur besides a sigmoid septum?

> ANS: There are several theories.
>
> > a. It is due to fibrosis, thickening, and often some calcification involving the bases of the aortic cusps. They do not open fully because of stiffness (aortic valve sclerosis). However, although they open enough to prevent any significant gradient across the orifice, there is enough narrowing to cause turbulence and an ejection murmur.
> >
> > b. It is due to calcific spurs on the aortic ring, which may protrude into the bloodstream.

A slight but abrupt protuberance (e.g. a calcium spur) is capable of producing a murmur of considerable intensity.

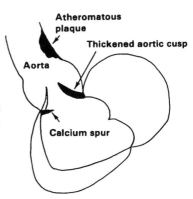

    c. It is due to atherosclerotic plaques in the ascending aorta, which may cause turbulence as the aortic stream strikes the roughened endocardium.

   Note: a. The general condition alluded to by these theories is called *aortic sclerosis.*

        b. If the valvular calcification that caused the sclerosis murmur becomes excessive, severe aortic valve obstruction may occur; this then becomes *calcific aortic stenosis.*

3. How loud can a murmur be that is due to aortic sclerosis?

   ANS: Up to grade 4/6.

4. What is the most important method of distinguishing by physical examination a loud murmur of aortic sclerosis from that of AS?

   ANS: Palpation of the carotid will generally differentiate between the slow rise of AS and the normal rise of aortic sclerosis. However, an elderly patient with significant AS may have a normal rate of rise if his or her carotids are sclerotic.

   Note: a. A reversed split S_2 in the absence of LBBB suggests a significant gradient. If the murmur is so loud and long that it is difficult to hear S_2 splitting clearly, use a pediatric diaphragm to soften the murmur.

        b. Bleeding from the right colon due to angiodysplasia occurs often enough in patients with AS to consider it a true association.

AORTIC STENOSIS EJECTION MURMURS _____

Valvular Aortic Stenosis Murmurs

Murmur Shape Duration and Quality

1. How can you tell the severity of aortic stenosis by the shape and length of the murmur?

   ANS: In general, the later the peak of the crescendo and the longer the murmur, the more severe is the stenosis.

2. How might the pitch and quality of an aortic ejection murmur sound at the apex? Why is this confusing? What is this phenomenon called?

   ANS: The high-frequency components tend to radiate to the apex and may even sound musical at this site suggesting a murmur of MR. This is called the Gallavardin phenomenon, which is especially common in the elderly patient, in whom the murmur of calcific AS often sounds musical or cooing at the apex. Commissural fusion is commonly absent in these valves, which allows the cusps to vibrate and produce pure frequencies.

3. What is the characteristic quality of the loud murmur of moderate to severe AS?

ANS: It tends to be harsh, rasping, grunting, and coarse, sounding like a person clearing his throat. This murmur can be imitated by placing your palm on the diaphragm of a stethoscope and listening through the earpiece while you scratch the dorsal surface of the hand with your fingernail.

Loudness and Site

1. Where is the aortic systolic murmur of valvular AS heard loudest?

ANS: Anywhere in a straight line from the second right interspace to the apex. (If the patient is obese or has emphysema, the murmur may be loudest above or on the clavicle.)

2. Where is the classic "aortic area?" What is wrong with this term?

ANS: This area is in the second right interspace. However, aortic valvular events can be best heard anywhere in a "sash" or "shoulder harness" area from the second right interspace to the apex.

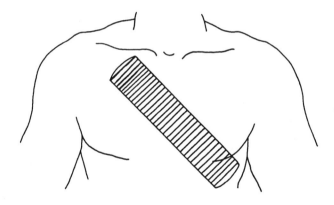

Aortic area

Since aortic ejection murmurs and clicks are often best heard at the apex area, and aortic regurgitation murmurs are usually best heard along the left lower sternal border or midsternum, it should no longer be taught that the "aortic area" is the second right interspace.

3. What term should we use instead of aortic area?

ANS: The second right interspace. It is confusing to a student to be told that aortic murmurs and ejection sounds are often best heard at the left sternal border or apex and then to hear the second right interspace called the aortic area.

4. What is characteristic of the upward radiation of an aortic murmur?

    ANS: a. It tends to radiate into the neck bilaterally but often radiates well along the innominate vein, making the murmur slightly louder on the left.

              b. It not only radiates well to the right clavicle but is usually amplified there. Any murmur louder over the carotid than on the clavicle should be considered a local arterial murmur [5].

    Note: Innocent aortic ejection murmurs are characteristically maximal along the left sternal border near the anatomical aortic valve area. With significant aortic valvular obstruction, however, the maximum turbulence occurs further downstream from the orifice and tends to be loudest at the second right interspace.

5. What is the significance of a soft A_2 in a patient with a loud ejection murmur?

    ANS: It almost always indicates severe AS because the soft A_2 implies heavy calcification of the valve.

6. How soft can the murmur of a severe AS become if heart failure develops with a resultant reduced stroke volume?

    ANS: It may almost disappear.

7. Why may the murmur of severe AS be soft in the elderly in the absence of heart failure?

    ANS: a. There is commonly an increased anteroposterior chest diameter in the elderly, especially at the base of the heart.

              b. The stiff cusp bases and lack of commissural fusion may cause some of the blood to be ejected between the cusps in the form of a "spray" rather than a jet. This may make the murmur not only more musical but also less loud and harsh.

Summary of Auscultatory Clues to the Diagnosis of Severe Aortic Stenosis

The AS is probably severe, i.e., the gradient is at least 70 mm Hg, or in the presence of congestive heart failure at least 50 mm Hg, if:

1. An S_4 is present in a patient under age 40.

2. The murmur is long with its peak in mid-systole, is at least grade 4/6, and is associated with a soft or absent A_2.

3. The S_2 has a reversed split provided there is no marked poststenotic dilatation to further delay the A_2.

    Note: The area of the normally open aortic valve is 3–4 cm². Symptoms usually do not develop until the area is reduced to about a third of normal or 1–1.5 cm², and patients even with this degree of narrowing may remain asymptomatic for decades. Some are symptom-free with orifices of 0.5 cm².

Hypertrophic Obstructive Cardiomyopathy (HOCM) Murmurs, or Hypertrophic Subaortic Stenosis (HSS)

1. What causes the obstruction in hypertrophic obstructive cardiomyopathy (HOCM)?

   ANS: The obstruction is usually caused by the combination of a hypertrophied septum, which bulges into the LV outflow tract during systole, and an abnormal anterior motion of the anterior leaflet of the mitral valve. The outflow tract, which is the space between the septum and the anterior leaflet of the mitral valve, becomes narrowed when a freely mobile portion of distal mitral valve is pulled toward the septum by a **Bernoulli effect**.

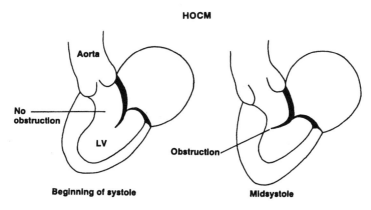

The asymmetric septal hypertrophy of the LV (known also as ASH) causes obstruction when the upper part of the septum meets a mobile part of the septal leaflet that is "sucked anteriorly." It is made mobile by an abnormal apposition of the anterior to the posterior leaflet.

   Note: a. Occasionally, even a distal portion of posterior leaflet can swing forward to cause obstruction to outflow.
   b. All patients with significant outflow tract obstruction have some MR by Doppler studies.

2. In HOCM, when in systole does the obstruction begin?

   ANS: Just prior to mid-systole.

3. When does the ejection murmur begin in HOCM?

   ANS: The murmur usually begins early because even though the obstruction is delayed to slightly beyond the time of onset of aortic valve opening, the tremendously rapid early ejection characteristic of HOCM can cause early turbulence. In the normal heart only about 50% of ventricular volume is ejected during the first half of systole, but in HOCM 80% or more is ejected during this period [6].

4. How can raising the blood pressure by a vasopressor agent or by having the patient squat help to differentiate between the ejection murmur of valvular AS and that of HOCM?

   ANS: A vasopressor agent will produce a bradycardia by the vagal effect of suddenly raising blood pressure. The bradycardia gives more time for diastolic filling, which will increase the volume and make the murmur of valvular AS louder. However, in HOCM the increase in pressure against the mitral leaflet will push the leaflet away from the septum and decrease the loudness of the murmur.

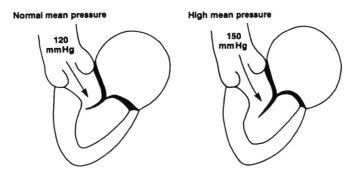

A high pressure in the aorta during ejection is transmitted to the mobile portion of the mitral valve leaflet and pushes it away from the septum and decreases the outflow obstruction.

5. What tends to make an HOCM obstruction worse, making the LV cavity smaller or making it larger? Why?

   ANS: Making it smaller allows the hypertrophied septum to obliterate the outflow tract space more easily.

6. How can a Valsalva maneuver help to differentiate the ejection murmur of valvular AS from that of HOCM?

   ANS: During the Valsalva maneuver the venous return is decreased, thus decreasing the stroke volume and the ejection murmur of valvular AS.

However, in a patient with HOCM, the decreased venous return produces a smaller LV and therefore more obstruction and a louder murmur.

Note: The Valsalva maneuver may not always work, because the obstruction may already be so severe that the Valsalva maneuver cannot produce any significant increase in obstruction.

7. How can amyl nitrite inhalation differentiate the ejection murmur of valvular AS from that of HOCM?

ANS: The blood pressure will drop immediately with amyl nitrite inhalation, but flow does not increase until about 20 s later. Therefore, the murmur of valvular AS, which is dependent on flow, will not begin to increase for about 20 s. The murmur of HOCM, on the other hand, will become louder within a few beats after inhalation, because as soon as the blood pressure drops (which occurs almost immediately), the loss of resistance to outflow causes a loss of support for the anterior leaflet of the mitral valve as the ventricle contracts. (See Chapter 14 for the hemodynamic effects of amyl nitrite.)

8. How will squatting differentiate between the murmur of HOCM and that of valvular AS?

ANS: Squatting, especially for the first few beats, will diminish the murmur of HOCM because it causes both increased venous return for a few beats and then a persistent increase in peripheral arterial resistance. In the presence of valvular AS, the increase in venous return will tend to increase the murmur.

Note: a. In standing after squatting, the systolic murmur sometimes doubles in intensity. The second or third repetition of squatting and standing may show more changes than first trial of squatting and standing.
   b. The physician should sit with the patient standing facing him. The patient should support himself or herself by a hand on the examining bed.
   c. In patients unable to squat, similar circulatory changes can be induced by bending the patient's knees on his abdomen while supine.
   d. The increased peripheral resistance on squatting is probably due to "kinking" of the femoral arteries as well as some isometric contraction effect.

9. What is peculiar about the site of greatest loudness of the HOCM murmur that may help to differentiate it from the murmur of valvular AS?

ANS: It is usually loudest near the apex, but occasionally it is loudest at the left lower sternal border.

Note: a. When septal hypertrophy is so great that it also produces RV outflow (infundibular) obstruction (rare), the murmur may be louder at the base than elsewhere (as in other forms of pulmonic stenosis).

b. The term asymmetric septal hypertrophy of the heart is often used to describe the heart in HOCM because the septum is dispro-portionately hypertrophied in relation to the hypertrophy of the free wall.

10. Why is there usually some MR with HOCM?

ANS: The hypertrophied septum may distort the direction in which the papillary muscles pull on the cusps.

Note: a. Mitral valve prolapse may occur in as many as 75% of patients with HOCM.

b. Occasionally a short apical early to mid-diastolic low-frequency murmur may be heard in HOCM, simulating mitral stenosis.

Supravalvular Aortic Stenosis Murmurs

1. List the clinical findings in supravalvular AS.

ANS: a. Peculiar "elfin" facies in the nonfamilial type (see Chapter 2 for facies of supravalvular AS).

b. Pulse volume greater in the right than in the left carotid and blood pressure higher in the right arm (see Chapter 3 for explanation).

c. No ejection sound, and a slight AR murmur.

d. The murmur may be loudest in the first right intercostal space.

Discrete Subvalvular Aortic Stenosis

1. What should make you suspect discrete subvalvular AS, i.e., an obstructive membrane or fibromuscular tunnel just below the aortic valve, as a cause of AS?

ANS: The absence of an ejection sound in the presence of an AR murmur in a young subject with no calcium in the aortic valve on echocardiogram or X-ray.

PULMONARY STENOSIS EJECTION MURMURS _____

1. Where is the classic "pulmonary area"? What is wrong with this term?

ANS: The classic pulmonary area is the second left interspace. Pulmonary events, however, may be best heard *anywhere* along the left sternal border (or even in the epigastrium in patients with chronic obstructive pulmonary disease).

2. Where is the best place for hearing the murmur of (a) valvular PS and (b) infundibular PS?

ANS: a. Valvular PS: best at the second left interspace.

       b. Infundibular PS: best at the third or fourth left interspace.

3. What is the relation between the peak of the crescendo of the PS murmur and the severity of the obstruction?

    ANS: The later the peak, the more severe is the obstruction.

4. Why is it that while in AS the murmur rarely peaks much beyond mid-systole, in PS the peak may go beyond mid-systole?

    ANS: The right ventricle (RV) is shaped like a teapot, with a main chamber, namely, the **inflow tract** (also known as the RV sinus), and a thick, high spout, which is the **outflow tract** or **infundibulum**.

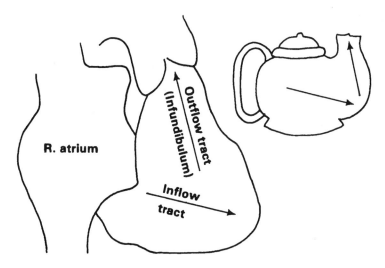

The outflow tract of the RV is a tubular structure made up mostly of muscle, called the crista supraventricularis, which separates the tricuspid from the pulmonary valves.

      The inflow and outflow tract contract asynchronously in a peristaltic fashion, the inflow tract first, then the infundibular or outflow tract. The worse the obstruction at the valve, the later the outflow tract contracts relative to the inflow tract [7]. It is the late contraction of this RV outflow tract that apparently produces the late peak of the crescendo.

      The LV, on the other hand, has no distinct muscular outflow tract. The anterior mitral leaflet and its chordae and papillary muscles form the posterolateral wall of a merely functional outflow tract, which is not anatomically independent enough to contract more than slightly asynchronously. (See figure on page 208.)

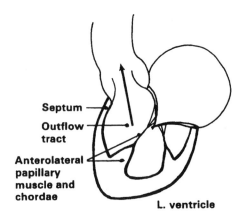

There is no infundibulum in the LV because the mitral and aortic valves are in direct continuity.

Septum

Outflow tract

Anterolateral papillary muscle and chordae

L. ventricle

The Murmur of Pulmonary Stenosis with Tetralogy of Fallot

1. What is meant by a severe **tetralogy of Fallot**?

    ANS: It refers to the presence of severe PS.

2. How does the severity of the PS affect the duration and loudness of the murmur in tetralogy? How does this differ from the PS murmur if the septum is intact?

    ANS: In tetralogy there are two outlets for RV ejection. Therefore, the greater the PS, the more goes out the aorta and the softer and shorter will be the ejection murmur. If the septum is intact, the greater the PS, the louder and longer is the murmur.

    Note: Amyl nitrite inhalation will soften the murmur of tetralogy but will increase the murmur of PS with an intact septum.

THE EFFECT OF RESPIRATION ON PS EJECTION MURMURS ___

1. Why may a PS ejection murmur not always increase during inspiration?

    ANS: Inspiration may place too much lung between the stethoscope and the heart, especially in the upper parasternal region (the basal area of the heart). Therefore, listen low on the chest or even posteriorly for the effect of inspiration.

2. Why does standing tend to exaggerate the increase in a PS murmur caused by inspiration?

    ANS: The increase in pulmonary flow caused by inspiration is about 15 mL whether the subject is lying down or standing. The total stroke volume, however, is decreased on standing by about 25% [8], so that the same 15-mL increase in stroke volume on inspiration is a proportionately larger amount of stroke volume ejected. Therefore, on standing there is a proportionately greater increase in gradient across the pulmonary valve.

3. How can a Valsalva maneuver distinguish a pulmonary ejection murmur from an aortic ejection murmur?

    ANS: During the strain phase, the decreased venous return causes all ejection murmurs (with the rare exception of the HSS murmur) to diminish. When the strain is released, the maximal loudness of the pulmonary ejection murmur will return immediately, i.e., within two or three beats. The maximal loudness of the aortic murmur will, however, be delayed for about six to ten beats owing to the time needed for the dammed-up venous blood to pass through the lungs to the LV and the aorta.

Summary of How to Distinguish a Pulmonary from an Aortic Stenosis Murmur by Auscultation

1. The AS murmur decreases slightly on inspiration. The PS murmur increases on inspiration, especially on standing and if you listen low on the chest and also posteriorly.

2. An AS murmur may be maximal in the second right intercostal space or near the apex. The PS murmur will only be maximal somewhere along the left sternal border.

3. The post-Valsalva effect causes an immediate return of loudness of the PS murmur but a delay in the return of loudness of the AS murmur.

4. If an ejection click is present, it will decrease or disappear on inspiration only with PS.

5. A wide, normally moving split S_2 with a soft second component (P_2) following the murmur indicates a murmur of PS rather than of AS.

THORACIC, SUBCLAVIAN, CAROTID, AND THYROID ARTERY FLOW MURMURS _____

1. What is characteristic of the timing and duration of a physiological (non-obstructive) vascular murmur?

    ANS: They are early in systole and short.

2. What are the characteristics of an arterial murmur due to obstruction?

    ANS: If a pressure difference across the obstruction is present in both systole and diastole, the murmur will be continuous, and the systolic murmur is always louder than the diastolic. The murmurs will have a mid- or late systolic peak if the obstruction is severe.

3. What is the difference between a bruit and a murmur?

   ANS: The word *bruit* (pronounced "broo-ee") is French for "noise" or "sound." In France, the first and second heart sounds are the first and second bruits. Our S_1 and S_2 are their B_1 and B_2. We misuse the word to mean an arterial murmur.

4. Which arterial flow murmur may cause an ejection type of murmur at the second right or left interspace?

   ANS: Rapid flow through the proximal branches of the aorta in young people. This is often mistaken for an aortic ejection murmur.

   Note: A carotid murmur is present in about 80% of children up to 4 years old but is found in only 10% of those in the older age groups.

5. How can you differentiate the supraclavicular arterial murmur of childhood from a basal valvular murmur?

   ANS: a. It is an arterial murmur unless it is louder on the clavicle than above it. Aortic valvular murmurs tend to be amplified on the clavicle.
   b. If the arm flow is increased by a hand-clenching exercise, only the arterial murmur will become louder.
   c. If the arm is stretched downward and backward, the subclavian artery is compressed between the clavicle and the first rib and the arterial murmur will diminish.
   d. Compress the subclavian artery with your finger, and note how the murmur changes with varying degrees of obstruction.

   Note: Listen also for a venous hum and an S_3 to confirm the presence of a hyperkinetic circulation. (See Chapter 14 for a method of eliciting a venous hum.)

6. What kind of peripheral arterial murmurs are heard in **coarctation**?

   ANS: Over the large collaterals of the back there are systolic flow murmurs with delayed onset (due to the time required for the systolic flow to reach the vessel and therefore continue beyond the S_2).

   Note: a. When the intercostals are collaterals, they become tortuous. Tortuosity creates turbulence.
   b. The murmur overlying the coarctation can be systolic or continuous, depending on the degree of aortic narrowing. The relatively high frequency requires the stethoscopic diaphragm.

7. What kind of murmur over the thyroid is heard in hyperthyroid patients?

   ANS: The arterial murmur is systolic. If a continuous murmur is heard, it is a venous hum.

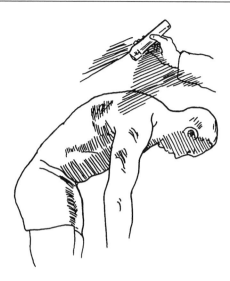

In the proper light, the dilated subcostal
collateral arteries can be seen to pulsate.

8. What is the timing, intensity, and site of the systolic murmur often heard after
   aortic coronary bypass surgery?

   ANS: It is a short, early ejection murmur not much more than grade 2/6, best
   heard when the patient is sitting up and leaning forward with held expiration. It is usually localized to the left sternal border and is usually
   heard only when the aortic coronary bypass is to the anterior descending artery.

   Note: When the murmur disappears, the bypass has often been found to be
   occluded, but not necessarily [9]. When present, the graft is patent. Dimi-
   nution with time may reflect a change from turbulent to laminar flow.

REFERENCES

1. Groom, D., et al. The normal systolic murmur. *Ann. Intern. Med.* 52:134, 1960.
2. Lessof, M., and Brigden, W. Systolic murmurs in healthy children and in children
   with rheumatic fever. *Lancet* 2:673,1967.
3. Dawson, A. A., and Palmer, K. N. V. The significance of cardiac murmurs in anemia.
   Am. J. Med. Sci. 25:554, 1966.
4. Perez, G. L., et al. Incidence of murmurs in the aging heart. *J. Am. Geriatr. Soc.*
   24:29, 1976.

5. Spodick, D. H., et al. Clavicular auscultation: Preferential clavicular transmission and amplification of aortic valve murmurs. *Chest* 70:337, 1976.

6. Pierce. G. E., Morrow, A. G., and Braunwald, E. Idiopathic hypertrophic subaortic stenosis. *Circulation* (Suppl. 4) 30:152, 1964.

7. Johnson. A. M. Functional infundibular stenosis, its differentiation from structural stenosis and its importance in atrial septal defect. *Guys Hosp. Rep.* 108:373, 1959.

8. Lewis. M. L., and Christianson, L. C. Effects of posture on lung blood volume in intact man. *Circulation* (Abstracts) (Suppl. III) 55 and 56:74, 1977.

9. Karpman, L. The murmur of aortocoronary bypass. *Am. Heart J.* 83:179 1972.

14 Systolic Regurgitant Murmurs

1. What is meant by a systolic regurgitant murmur?

   ANS: This is a murmur produced by retrograde flow from a high pressure area of the heart through some abnormal opening into an area of lower pressure.

2. What are the two abnormal openings that allow systolic regurgitation, besides the mitral and tricuspid valves?

   ANS: a. A **ventricular septal defect** (VSD) (high-pressure left ventricle, [LV] to low-pressure right ventricle [RV]).
   b. An arteriovenous communication such as persistent ductus arteriosus (PDA) (high-pressure area aorta to low-pressure pulmonary artery).

3. What characteristics are common to all systolic regurgitant murmurs?

   ANS: a. If there are early components, they start with the first heart sound. If there are late components, they always extend to or beyond the second heart sound of the same side.
   b. When soft, they are predominantly high-pitched and blowing because the opening is probably very small, and there is usually a high **gradient** between a ventricle and any chamber into which retrograde flow occurs.
   c. They tend to remain the same after sudden long diastoles. (For rare exceptions to this rule, see below.)

4. How can you imitate various kinds of high-pitched blowing murmurs?

   ANS: a. Whisper a drawn-out "haaa" or "hoo."
   b. Say a drawn-out "shsh" or "ffff."
   c. Hold the diaphragm of the stethoscope against the palm of your hand and listen through the earpieces while you run the pads of your fingers across the back of your hand.

5. What are regurgitant murmurs called if they stretch from the S_1 to the S_2?

   ANS: Pansystolic or holosystolic murmurs.

Boldface type indicates that the term is explained in the glossary.

6. When does a systolic regurgitant murmur become a continuous murmur?

    ANS: If it extends far enough beyond the S_2 to be recognized by the listener as reaching into diastole.

THE EFFECT OF A SUDDEN LONG DIASTOLE ON LEFT-SIDED REGURGITANT MURMURS _____

1. What will happen to the loudness of a left-sided regurgitant murmur, such as that heard in mitral regurgitation (MR) or VSD, after a sudden long diastole?

    ANS: The loudness usually remains about the same. (Listening for the effect of a sudden long diastole is one of best ways to differentiate an ejection from a regurgitant murmur.)

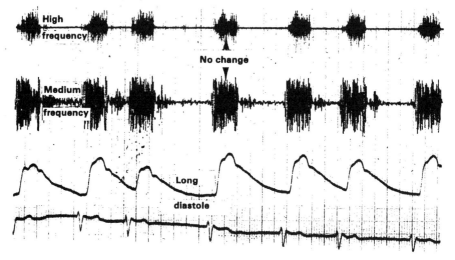

A high- and medium-frequency phonocardiogram taken at the apex together with an external carotid tracing from a 45-year-old woman with moderately severe chronic rheumatic MR, with few symptoms on digitalis alone. Because of atrial fibrillation, short and long diastoles are present, demonstrating that the murmur does not grow louder after long diastoles than after short or average diastoles.

    Note: If the pause is caused by a premature ventricular contraction (PVC), compare the postextrasystolic beat not with the PVC but with the normal cycle following the postextrasystolic beat. A PVC may be so premature that there is no time for any significant ventricular filling. Therefore, the loudness of a murmur produced by the PVC itself is of no significance.

2. Why does the left-sided regurgitant murmur not usually become louder despite a larger volume in the ventricle after a sudden long diastole, as after a PVC?

    ANS: In MR, VSD, and PDA, the LV has two outlets during systole. The amount ejected through each outlet depends on the relative resistance beyond each outlet. During the PVC, the aortic pressure is less than normal because of the small stroke volume. During the long diastole after the PVC, the pressure beyond the aortic outlet falls still more, owing to continued long runoff into the periphery. Thus, by the time of the next systole the resistance at the aortic valve has dropped so low that blood is preferentially ejected into the aorta, and relatively less is regurgitated through the other orifice. One would think at first that this would make the murmur softer. However, because there is more volume in the LV at the end of a long diastole, the absolute quantity of blood regurgitated remains about the same as that after short diastoles.

3. When may the MR murmur become softer after a long diastole?

    ANS: a. In the prolapsed mitral valve syndrome. (See the section on prolapsed mitral valve syndrome for explanation, p. 225).

    b. In some papillary muscle dysfunction murmurs, when myocardial ischemia rather than fibrosis causes the MR [1]. The long diastole may decrease myocardial ischemia by allowing more time for coronary filling and by decreasing the afterload due to the increased time allowed for aortic pressure to fall.

MITRAL REGURGITATION MURMURS _____

Terminology

1. Why may it be preferable to use the term *mitral regurgitation* rather than *mitral incompetence* or *mitral insufficiency*, even though cardiologists are about equally divided as to the preferred usage?

    ANS: The abbreviation for mitral incompetence or insufficiency is MI, which is also used as an abbreviation for myocardial infarction. There is no confusion when MR is used.

    Note: Regurgitation describes the direction of the flow, whereas incompetence or insufficiency describes the condition of the valve. For the sake of consistency, we shall use the terms aortic, pulmonary, and tricuspid regurgitation, instead of incompetence or insufficiency.

Causes

1. List the four most common causes of MR murmurs in the adult.

   ANS: Prolapse of the mitral leaflet into the left atrium, papillary muscle dysfunction, rheumatic valve damage, and ruptured chordae.

   Note: When a loud S_1 is heard in a patient with MR, mitral valve prolapse should be considered.

2. List some rare causes of MR in the adult.

   ANS: Left atrial myxoma, an endocardial cushion defect with a cleft anterior leaflet, and a calcified mitral annulus.

   Note: About 10% of patients with mitral annulus calcification have severe MR [2].

3. What are the usual causes of papillary muscle dysfunction murmurs?

   ANS: Myocardial infarction, recent or old, with or without a ventricular aneurysm and with or without papillary muscle fibrosis. Infarction of the ventricle at the base of the papillary muscles or ischemia of that area of the ventricle, which may occur with an attack of angina may cause marked MR even with a normal papillary muscle.

   Note: About 10% of papillary muscle dysfunction murmurs that are due to acute infarction will disappear before the patient leaves the hospital [3].

Loudness, Sites, and Radiation of Mitral Regurgitation Murmurs

1. Where are MR murmurs loudest?

   ANS: At the apex area or slightly lateral to the site of the apex impulse.

2. Where is the best radiation zone of the usual MR murmur?

   ANS: It usually radiates best to the axilla and the left posterior intrascapular area of the chest. However, if loud enough, it will radiate to the right, but to a lesser degree.

   Note: When the murmur is due to ruptured chordae, it may have an unusual radiation zone. (See Questions 3 and 4 under MR Due to Ruptured Chordae.)

3. Besides an obese or emphysematous chest, what can cause severe MR to be silent?

   ANS: a. Prosthetic MR due to suture breakdown.
   b. Papillary muscle rupture during acute infarction.

   Note: Soft MR murmurs can disappear during pregnancy due to the peripheral vasodilation and fall in systemic resistance.

Shape, Pitch, and Duration of Mitral Regurgitation Murmurs

1. What are all the possible shapes of an MR murmur?

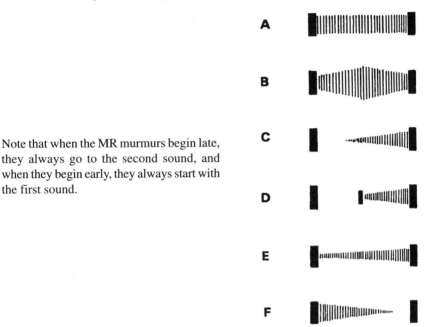

Note that when the MR murmurs begin late, they always go to the second sound, and when they begin early, they always start with the first sound.

2. What shape are the loudest MR murmurs?

   ANS: Pansystolic and slightly crescendo–decrescendo. The crescendo–decrescendo shape in these patients is better described as a spindle shape on a phonocardiogram.

3. How does the pitch of a murmur correlate with gradient and flow?

   ANS: High gradients and little flow produce high-pitched murmurs. High flow and low gradients produce low-pitched murmurs.

4. Which MR murmurs are always associated with almost pure high frequencies, i.e., only a blowing sound?

   ANS: All soft murmurs with small volume flows and high gradients, e.g., those due to trivial MR.

   Note: The gradient between the left atrium and LV usually reaches more than 100 mmHg during the peak of systole.

5. Why does the MR murmur extend slightly beyond the S_2?

   ANS: Because LV pressure is higher than left atrial pressure even after the aortic valve closes. (See figure on p. 218.)

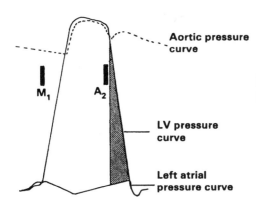

Aortic pressure curve

M_1 A_2

Note that the LV pressure is above left atrial pressure, even after the A_2.

LV pressure curve

Left atrial pressure curve

6. Is an MR murmur louder on inspiration or expiration?

ANS: It is usually louder on expiration because that is when blood is pushed into the LV from the lungs.

Quantitating the Degree of Mitral Regurgitation

1. How can you tell the degree of MR by palpation?

ANS: The MR is greater:

   a. The larger the LV by palpation.
   b. The greater and later the left parasternal movement. (This may represent the left atrium expanding during systole.)
   c. The more palpable an early rapid filling wave and S_3 at the apex.

2. How can you tell the degree of MR by auscultation?

ANS: The MR is greater:

   a. The louder and longer the apical systolic murmur. However, although ruptured chordae murmurs may be decrescendo, they are almost always at least grade 3/6 in loudness [4].
   b. The louder the S_3, since this is roughly proportional to the torrential diastolic flow, with the exception of sudden severe MR due to ruptured chordae on a previously normal mitral valve. The S_3 here is either soft or absent.
   c. The longer and louder the diastolic flow murmur following the S_3. (See figure on p. 219.)
   d. The wider the split of the S_2, unless the development of severe pulmonary hypertension narrows the split.

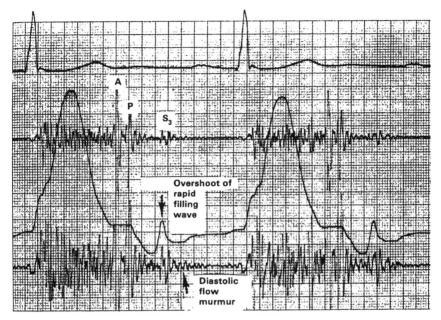

This phonocardiogram and apical pulse tracing is from a 15-year-old girl with severe rheumatic MR. The pulse tracing was taken over the LV impulse in the supine position and is therefore an apex precordiogram instead of an apex cardiogram, which is taken in the left lateral decubitus position. The phonocardiograms are from the third left parasternal interspace. The upper one is taken at medium frequency; the lower one brings out low and medium frequencies. Note the following signs of severe MR: (1) the widely split S_2 of 50 ms; (2) the diastolic flow murmur after the S_3; (3) the exaggerated early rapid filling peak of the apical impulse (this would be palpable in the left lateral decubitus position).

Papillary Muscle Dysfunction Murmurs

1. How can different kinds of papillary muscle dysfunction produce MR murmurs of different shapes?

   ANS: a. If, when the ventricle contracts, one papillary muscle is unable to contract or is attached to infarcted muscle at its base, the papillary muscle and its chordae will be longer than the opposite normally contracting papillary muscle and its chordae. As the systolic pressure rises and the LV cavity decreases in size, the portion of the mitral leaflets with the relatively long papillary muscle and its chordae will project more and more into the left atrium, producing a crescendo murmur to the S_2. (See figures on p. 220.)

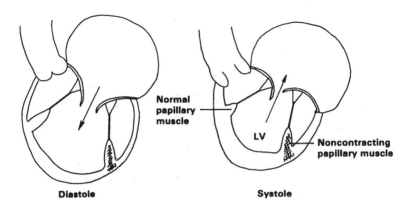

Diastole   Systole

A noncontracting papillary muscle may make its chordae-plus-papillary muscle relatively longer as the ventricle becomes smaller. This is most likely to produce a murmur that becomes progressively louder as systole proceeds (crescendo murmur to the S_2).

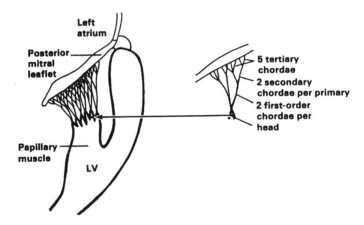

b. Fixed shortening of a papillary muscle by marked fibrosis or by attachment to an aneurysmal or dilated akinetic area will cause pansystolic regurgitation.

c. The murmur may be decrescendo if dilatation is the major cause of the regurgitation.

2. How does the presence of an S_4 help tell you the etiology of an MR murmur?

   ANS: If an S_4 is present, it strongly suggests papillary muscle dysfunction secondary to a **cardiomyopathy**. Rheumatic MR is rarely associated with an S_4.

   Note: The degree of MR after infarction is greater for posterior than for anterior infarction.

MR Due to a Ruptured Papillary Muscle

1. How many chordae are capable of rupture if a papillary muscle ruptures?

    ANS: Each papillary muscle has about six heads whose chordae divide about three times before they attach to their leaflets, to each of which are attached about 120 tertiary chordae. (See figures on p. 220.)

2. What is the usual cause of a papillary muscle rupture?

    ANS: Myocardial infarction.

3. How may loudness of the murmur tell you whether a systolic regurgitant apical area murmur is due to a ruptured papillary muscle rather than to a ventricular septal rupture?

    ANS: With a ruptured papillary muscle the regurgitation is so severe that together with the myocardial damage of the infarction the murmur rarely exceeds grade 3/6, i.e., it is rare to feel a thrill with it. Occasionally, profound MR can exist with only faint systolic murmurs. Ventricular septal ruptures are usually loud enough to have a thrill.

MR Due to Ruptured Chordae

1. How does spontaneous rupture differ from that due to **infective endocarditis**?

    ANS: Spontaneous ruptures usually occur in one of the 25 major chordae closer to the papillary muscles than to the leaflets, thus involving at least four or five small terminal branches. Infective endocarditis usually involves only a few terminal branches.

2. What is the shape and frequency of the usual MR murmur of spontaneously ruptured chordae? Why?

    ANS: It is a decrescendo, mixed-frequency murmur. It is decrescendo because the left atrium does not enlarge much with acute severe MR, due to the nondistensible pericardium around the atria. This poor left atrial compliance may raise the V-wave pressure to a very high peak as high as 70 mmHg toward the end of systole). The rise in left atrial pressure plus a precipitous fall in LV pressure toward the end of systole decreases the end-systolic gradient and murmur. (See figure on p. 222.)

3. Why may ruptured chordae imitate aortic stenosis (AS)?

    ANS: If posterior chordae rupture, producing a flail posterior cusp, the stream of regurgitation may strike the atrial septum in such a way that it can generate murmurs with the shape and radiation into the carotids that are typical of those seen with AS murmurs.

    Note: Despite good radiation into the second right interspace and neck, the murmur of a posterior chordae rupture is still usually loudest at the apex.

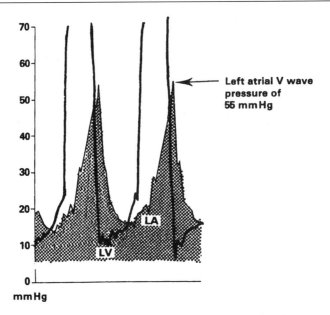

This is a left atrial (wedge) and LV pressure tracing from a 23-year-old woman with ruptured mitral chordae. The shaded area is under the left atrial (wedge) pressure curve. The slight delay in the peak wedge pressure is due to the fact that wedge pressures (taken by a catheter wedged into the distal pulmonary arterial branches) always show a delay in comparison with direct left atrial pressure tracings. The rapid increase in V-wave pressure during systole rapidly decreases the gradient across the mitral valve and will tend to cause both a decrescendo gradient and murmur. The decompressing effect on the LV of the massive loss of blood into the left atrium causes a late systolic fall in LV pressure. This end-systolic decrease in LV pressure further decreases the gradient across the mitral valve toward the end of systole.

4. What is the characteristic radiation of an MR murmur caused by rupture of the anterior chordae?

   ANS: It may radiate along the spine and if loud, even to the top of the head. See illustration on p. 223.

5. Which diastolic sound tells you that a loud MR murmur is due to ruptured chordae rather than to rheumatic heart disease?

   ANS: The healthy atrial wall resists acute dilatation in patients with ruptured chordae. It responds to the stretch produced by the massive regurgitant stream with a **Starling effect**, and by contracting strongly it often produces an S_4, which is rare in rheumatic MR.

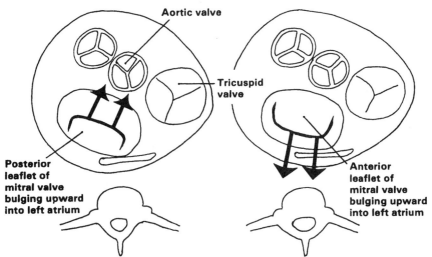

These views of the valve rings from above show how posterior ruptured chordae (on left) can direct the regurgitant stream against the aorta and cause the murmur to be transmitted like an aortic ejection murmur. The diagram at right shows how ruptured anterior chordae can direct the regurgitant stream posteriorly against the spine.

6. What are the usual causes of ruptured chordae?

   ANS: Infective endocarditis on either a rheumatic or a prolapsed myxomatous mitral valve. Often a prolapse has been present for years before the rupture but has not been recognized as such.

7. What most closely imitates the auscultatory findings of ruptured chordae?

   ANS: A severe form of prolapsed mitral valve with marked mysomatous degeneration. This is known as the *floppy valve syndrome*.

   Note: Most mitral valves are removed or repaired because of mitral regurgitation due to severe prolapse.

EFFECT OF DRUGS AND MANEUVERS ON SYSTOLIC REGURGITANT MURMURS _____

Raising Peripheral Resistance or Blood Volume

1. What happens to left-sided regurgitant murmurs if the peripheral resistance is increased? Why?

   ANS: They become louder, because with regurgitation there are two outlets for systole, and an increased resistance at the aortic outlet promotes more outflow through the regurgitant outlet.

2. How will raising the blood pressure with handgrip, squatting, or phenylephrine help you to determine whether a long systolic murmur at the apex is due to AS or MR?

   ANS: With increased peripheral resistance, aortic ejection murmurs will either be unchanged or become softer, but MR murmurs will become louder.

Decreasing Peripheral Resistance with Nitrites

1. How does amyl nitrite affect blood pressure and cardiac output? How do its effects differ from those of nitroglycerin?

   ANS: Amyl nitrite causes an immediate and marked drop in blood pressure. After about 20 s the cardiac output is increased. Nitroglycerin causes a mild drop in blood pressure and a fall in cardiac output.

2. Why does amyl nitrite cause an increase in cardiac output whereas nitroglycerin causes a fall in cardiac output?

   ANS: The rapid and profound drop in blood pressure produced by amyl nitrite results in a strong reflex sympathetic outflow that constricts the veins. Amyl nitrite is volatile and is dissipated in the capillary system before it reaches the veins. The direct effect of amyl nitrite on the capillaries may open up shunts between the dilated arterioles and venules. The increased venous return, together with the reflex tachycardia, increases the cardiac output. Nitroglycerin, on the other hand, does affect the veins and reduces venous return by causing venous pooling.

3. How can amyl nitrite help to separate an aortic ejection murmur from an MR murmur at the apex?

   ANS: By decreasing the peripheral resistance, it makes the MR murmur softer. By causing an increased velocity of ejection through the aortic valve, it makes the aortic ejection murmur louder.

   Note: A marked effect may be achieved with only three inhalations of amyl nitrite. The following precautions are helpful when using amyl nitrite:
   a. Wear rubber gloves, or the odor may remain on your fingers for days.
   b. Never use it unless the patient is supine, or you may produce syncope.
   c. Warn the patient that he will feel flushed and that his or her heart will pound for about 30 s.
   d. An assistant should call out the systolic blood pressures throughout the entire procedure so that you will know whether and to what degree the blood pressure is affected.

THE PROLAPSED MITRAL VALVE SYNDROME (BARLOW'S SYNDROME) _____

Definitions and Terminology

1. What is meant by a ballooned or prolapsed mitral valve? What auscultatory findings does it cause?

    ANS: This term refers to the bulging or buckling of one or both mitral valve leaflets into the left atrium during systole, so that one or more crisp systolic sounds or clicks and a late systolic MR murmur are commonly heard. The systolic murmur usually goes to the A_2. There may be only a click, only a murmur, or both.

2. How common are prolapsed mitral valves in asymptomatic subjects?

    ANS: About 2% of asymptomatic women age 18–35 years have prolapse by echo screening.

3. How has the term *floppy valve* been misused?

    ANS: The term *floppy valve syndrome* has been applied by some as a synonym for the prolapsed valve syndrome. This is unfortunate, because this term was originally meant to describe the most marked degree of myxomatous degeneration; causing severe MR. In the usual prolapsed valve syndrome, the MR is at most only moderate.

4. What can we call the click or sound that often precedes the delayed systolic murmur?

    ANS: A nonejection click or sound. It cannot be called mid-systolic, because at times it may come as early as an ejection click and as late as a widely split S_2.

    Note: a. Multiple clicks are common.
    b. If the etiology is primarily myocardial infarction and papillary muscle dysfunction, it is not so likely to sound like a click.

Etiology, Pathology, and Physiology of the Prolapsed Valve Syndrome

1. What is the usual mitral valve abnormality seen at surgery or necropsy when a prolapsed mitral valve is examined?

    ANS: Myxomatous transformation with elongated chordae. (See figure on p. 226.)

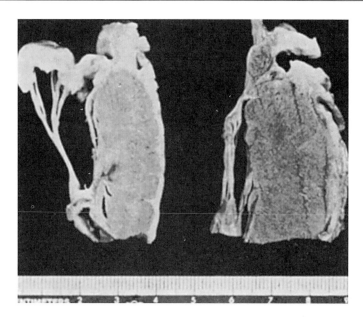

On the left is a cross section of the abnormal middle scallop of the posterior leaflet. On the right is the same area from a woman with left ventricular hypertrophy but no MR. (From J. K. Trent, et al. *Am. Heart J.* 79:539, 1970.)

2. With what conditions have prolapsed valves been most commonly associated?

   ANS: a. The **Marfan syndrome**.
         b. Papillary muscle dysfunction due to myocardial infarction.
         c. **Hypertrophic obstructive cardiomyopathy** (HOCM).
         d. **Atrial septal defects** (ASDs).

3. What is the cause of the nonejection click preceding the delayed systolic murmur?

   ANS: The "chordal snap" theory contends that the click is due to a sudden stretch of chordae as they give way with the peak pressure in midsystole. However, because the papillary muscles contract early, the chordae are under too much tension from the beginning of systole to "snap" during ventricular ejection. Therefore, this theory has been challenged by another theory that suggests that the click is a *valvular* sound produced by the loss of support of one leaflet by its opposing leaflet due to redundant valve tissue or to an abnormality of chordal length [5]. Thus, a small piece of unsupported leaflet may suddenly flip upward to its full extent to produce a click.

   Note: a. Other causes of midsystolic clicks include a small left-sided pneumothorax, pleuro-pericardial adhesions, absent pericardium, and an aneurysm of the atrial septum or of the membranous ventricular septum, usually with a small VSD.

b. An early diastolic click may be heard in 5–15% of patients with MVP, due to reverse ballooning of the prolapsed mitral leaflets.

4. How much MR is present if a delayed murmur to the S_2 is present?

   ANS: Since there is little or no regurgitation at the beginning of systole in these patients, only a mild to moderate amount of MR is likely to be present with this kind of murmur.

5. What can cause the development of heart failure in a patient with mild MR secondary to the prolapsed valve syndrome, besides ruptured chordae?

   ANS: Infective endocarditis on the mitral valve can occur.

Prolapsed Valve Auscultatory Findings

Shape and Loudness of Click and Murmur

1. What is the usual shape of delayed systolic murmurs in prolapsed mitral valve syndrome?

   ANS: To the ear, they often sound crescendo to the second sound.

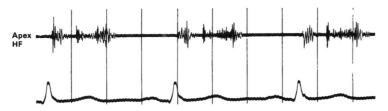

The midsystolic sound was a click heard loudest at the apex in this 45-year-old woman. The murmur following it is crescendo to the S_2. This is the classic ballooned valve click-murmur complex by auscultation.

2. What peculiar kind of murmur quality is almost pathognomonic of a prolapsed mitral valve?

   ANS: Systolic musical honks or whoops are not an uncommon sign of a prolapsed valve. They are usually transient and disappear with different phases of respiration. When they have disappeared, a regurgitant murmur is almost always present. (The word *honk* refers to the similarity of this sound to the honking of a goose.) These musical honks or whoops are the loudest murmurs heard in cardiologic practice. Many of these patients can hear their own murmurs, and some murmurs can even be heard across the room.

Note: Musical MR murmurs or honks are due to vibrations of the valves themselves [6]. The usual murmur is caused by turbulence around the valve rather than by the vibrations themselves.

Changing the Click and Murmur with Maneuvers or Drugs

1. What happens to the nonejection click and murmur when blood volume to the LV is decreased, as occurs with standing, inspiration, or a Valsalva strain?

    ANS: They both occur earlier and they often become louder. Indeed, they may be heard only on sitting or standing.

2. Why does the prolapsed valve murmur become louder and begin earlier on standing or with any maneuver that makes the heart smaller?

    ANS: Angiograms have shown that an increase in prolapse occurs in the upright position. This may occur because the redundant tissue acts like the dome of a parachute, whose diameter is decreased if the edges are held down and pulled toward each other. That is, when the ventricle becomes smaller and the diameter is reduced, the center of the "parachute" is pushed up, owing to the fixed length of chordae and papillary muscles in the smaller ventricle.

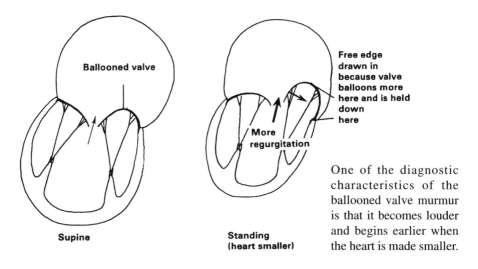

Balloooned valve

Free edge drawn in because valve balloons more here and is held down here

More regurgitation

Supine

Standing (heart smaller)

One of the diagnostic characteristics of the ballooned valve murmur is that it becomes louder and begins earlier when the heart is made smaller.

3. What maneuver can tell you that a crescendo systolic murmur to the S_2 is due to papillary muscle dysfunction rather than to the prolapsed valve syndrome if the latter happens to have no click?

    ANS: Only the prolapsed valve murmur will become louder and longer and begin earlier on sitting or standing.

4. How can you differentiate the late systolic murmur of papillary muscle dysfunction from the late systolic murmur of a prolapsed mitral valve (without a click) by auscultation?

    ANS: Papillary muscle dysfunction murmurs are usually associated with an S_4 and a loud S_1. They often become softer after a sudden long diastole, and increase with squatting or amyl nitrite. Prolapsed valve murmurs have no characteristic S_1, do not usually feature an S_4, and may become softer with squatting or amyl nitrite.

TRICUSPID REGURGITATION (TR) MURMURS _____

Site, Loudness, and Shape

1. Where is the murmur of TR usually heard best? In what other places may it occasionally be heard?

    ANS: It is usually heard best at the left lower sternal border. It is occasionally heard best in the epigastrium, at the right sternal border or, if the RV is very large, over the mid-left thorax at the site of the usual LV apex area, which may be taken over by the RV. When there is acute, severe TR, there may be no precordial regurgitant murmur; but the massive reflux into the venous system may produce a systolic murmur and thrill at the root of the neck.

2. What is the classic method of diagnosing TR by auscultation?

    ANS: Listen for a pansystolic murmur that becomes louder with inspiration at the left lower sternal border (or wherever a palpable RV lift is felt). This has been called the Carvallo sign of TR [7].

    Note: a. The murmur of TR remains louder on held inspiration (inspiratory apnea), i.e., it does not require moving respiration.

    b. Occasionally the TR murmur will not increase with inspiration, especially if the TR is severe or the RV fails so that the increase in RV volume cannot be converted into an increase in stroke volume.

3. How, besides by inspiration, can you increase venous return in order to bring out a TR murmur?

    ANS: a. By exercise.

    b. By having someone hold the patient's legs up or having the patient bend his or her knees up toward the chest.

    c. By amyl nitrite inhalation.

    d. By pressure over or just below the liver [8].

    e. Have patient stand suddenly. This will cause a momentary decrease in right-sided filling pressure, and respiration changes in venous return may become apparent.

Note: Severe TR can cause systolic expansion of the liver, which is elicited by placing the right hand on the right upper quadrant and pushing upward from behind with the left hand.

4. How can a Valsalva maneuver help to distinguish TR from MR on auscultation if the site of maximal loudness and the effect of respiration are questionable?

ANS: Upon release of the strain, the TR murmur returns to the pre-Valsalva level of loudness within about 1 s. An MR murmur should not return for at least about 3 s.

Note: Tricuspid regurgitation murmurs can become louder after a sudden long diastole, because the larger volume creates more regurgitation and pulmonary vascular resistance does not fall enough to increase forward flow more than regurgitant flow.

Causes of TR

1. Does a hypertrophied RV, due to high pressure within it (as in severe pulmonary stenosis or pulmonary hypertension) usually cause significant TR?

ANS: No. The TR thus caused is *secondary* TR. It requires both a high pressure and a large volume in the RV.

Note: Primary TR means TR occurring without pulmonary hypertension, such as that due to trauma, to **Ebstein's anomaly**, or to infective endocarditis. (The latter is seen primarily in heroin addicts.) Primary TR often results in an early systolic murmur.

2. What is the most common cause of both a high pressure and a large volume in the RV, so that TR is expected?

ANS: Severe pulmonary hypertension.

THE CARDIORESPIRATORY MURMUR _____

1. What is meant by a cardiorespiratory (or cardiopulmonary) murmur?

ANS: It is an extracardiac murmur, probably produced when the systolic motion of the heart compresses an expanded lung segment between the pericardium and the pleura.

2. What is the pitch and timing of this murmur?

ANS: It is high-pitched, usually short, and may occur anywhere in systole and even in early diastole. It is heard best during deep inspiration. It tends to disappear near the end of expiration and during held inspiration. It may mimic a late systolic MR murmur, a short aortic regurgitation (AR) murmur, a TR murmur, or a friction rub.

VSD MURMURS

Shapes and Length

1. Where is the usual VSD situated?

    ANS: In the membranous septum, i.e., in a small translucent area, extending
    about 1 or 2 cm below the aortic valve.

    Note: The attachment of the septal leaflet of the tricuspid valve bisects the
    membranous septum, so that the usual VSD is below the attachment,
    but if the VSD is above this attachment it may shunt blood directly into
    the right atrium.

Defects in the membranous septum
below the tricuspid valve are the
most common.

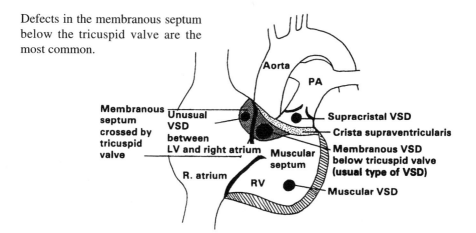

2. What are the various shapes of VSD murmurs?

    ANS:

Unlike some MR murmurs,
VSD murmurs probably always
begin with the M1.

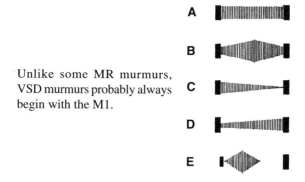

3. When is the VSD murmur mostly decrescendo?

   ANS: If it is of the muscular type, i.e., in the muscular part of the septum. Muscular contraction of the septum can close the VSD off toward the end of systole.

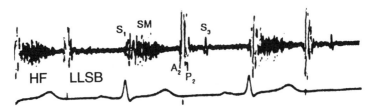

Small muscular VSD murmur in a 16-year-old girl. Her physiological S_3 is loud enough to be heard at the left lower sternal border (LLSB), probably because she has a long chest with a slightly medially placed apex beat.

4. How can you make the short decrescendo of a muscular VSD obviously pansystolic?

   ANS: By increasing peripheral resistance either by squatting, handgrip, or by using a vasopressor agent.

5. Why may a very large VSD produce a short ejection murmur or no murmur at all?

   ANS: It may create, in effect, a single ventricle, with the same systolic pressure in both RV and LV so that the shunt murmur may be soft or may even disappear. Thus, the systolic murmur that you hear may be only an ejection murmur due to flow into a slightly dilated pulmonary artery.

   Note: The syndrome of a VSD with pulmonary hypertension severe enough to cause a right-to-left shunt may be called **Eisenmenger's complex**, because this is what Eisenmenger originally described. If the right-to-left shunt is at PDA or ASD levels, it is called **Eisenmenger syndrome**.

Factors Controlling Loudness of VSD Murmurs

1. What is the relationship between the size of the VSD and the loudness of the murmur?

   ANS: If it is very small (pinhole VSD), the murmur may be very soft. If it is very large, so that there are almost equal pressures in the RV and the LV, the murmur may also be very soft. If, however, it is moderately large, there is usually a very loud murmur. (Some of the loudest murmurs observed in cardiological practice, next to prolapsed valve honks, are caused by moderately large VSDs.)

2. What auscultatory clues indicate that a soft VSD murmur is due to a large VSD with severe pulmonary hypertension?

   ANS: a. The murmur is often preceded by an ejection sound when the pulmonary artery is dilated.

   b. If a large flow is still present (the pulmonary hypertension is then said to be hyperkinetic, vasoactive, or vasospastic), a mitral diastolic murmur due to excess flow through the mitral valve may be heard.

Factors Controlling Sites of Loudness

1. What is the usual site of maximal loudness of the VSD murmur?

   ANS: The left lower sternal border.

2. When may a VSD murmur be louder between the apex and the left lower sternal border than at the left sternal border?

   ANS: When the VSD is in the muscular part of the septum near the apex. This is not an unusual site for a ruptured septum secondary to infarction.

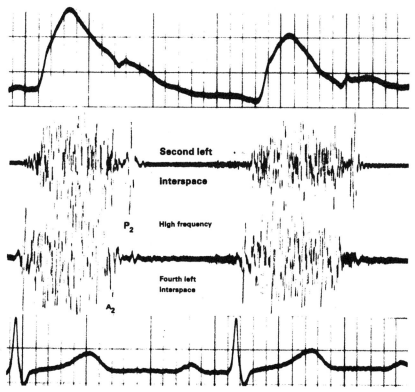

Loud pansystolic harsh murmur found in a patient with a large VSD.

3. What is meant by *maladie de Roger*?

    ANS: In 1861, the French pediatrician Henri Roger presented the first comprehensive description of an asymptomatic VSD and described the murmur through the defect as loud and long, with its maximum intensity over the upper third of the medial precordial area [9]. The expression is now used to refer to a small VSD with a loud murmur at the left lower sternal border. Roger, however, neither specified the size of the VSD nor placed the murmur at the lower sternal border.

The VSD Murmur Versus the MR Murmur

1. How can you tell by auscultation whether a pansystolic murmur that develops during acute infarction and is loudest near the apex is due to acute MR or is a VSD secondary to a ruptured septum?

    ANS: When the ventricular septum ruptures due to infarction it may do so in the muscle near the apex and mimic the site of the murmur of MR. However, this VSD murmur will be found to be louder slightly medial to the apex. (MR murmurs are usually loudest slightly lateral to the apex impulse.) Furthermore, papillary muscle ruptures very rarely have a grade 4/6 murmur, but about 50% of VSD murmurs commonly have this loud a murmur. Also, a VSD due to a ruptured septum commonly has a medium- to high-frequency presystolic murmur [10].

    Note: A windsock sound is a nonejection click associated with the sudden slapping motion of a ventricular septal aneurysm into the RV. It results in a widely split S_1.

CONTINUOUS MURMURS _____

Definitions and Causes

1. What are the two definitions of a continuous murmur?

    ANS: a. The murmur never stops, i.e. it is truly continuous throughout systole and diastole.

    b. The murmur can be heard to go beyond the S_2 but stops before the next S_1, i.e., it is not truly continuous but does envelop the second sound and goes more than slightly beyond it.

2. What is a systolic and diastolic murmur heard in the same area called if it is not continuous?

    ANS: A to-and-fro murmur. This implies that the systolic component is due to blood flowing in one direction and the diastolic murmur is due to flow in the opposite direction, e.g., an AS ejection murmur plus an AR murmur. A continuous murmur, on the other hand, implies a murmur that is due to continuous flow in the same direction in both systole and diastole.

3. Are all continuous murmurs regurgitant?

  ANS: No. Continuous murmurs may be caused by

  a. Partial obstruction to a vessel, as in bilateral peripheral pulmonary artery stenosis.

  b. Excessively rapid flow through tortuous vessels, as in collateral circulation secondary to a coarctation of the aorta.

  c. Extracardiac arterial or venous turbulence:

   (1) The mammary souffle (see below).

   (2) Bronchial collateral circulation in cyanotic congenital heart disease with severe obstruction to pulmonary arterial flow.

   (3) An arteriovenous fistula.

   (4) Total anomalous pulmonary venous connection (heard under either clavicle).

   (5) Across a small ASD with mitral stenosis (Lutembacher syndrome) or with MR (best in right third or fourth intercostal spaces).

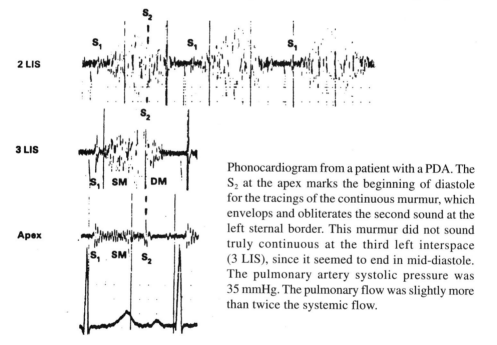

Phonocardiogram from a patient with a PDA. The S_2 at the apex marks the beginning of diastole for the tracings of the continuous murmur, which envelops and obliterates the second sound at the left sternal border. This murmur did not sound truly continuous at the third left interspace (3 LIS), since it seemed to end in mid-diastole. The pulmonary artery systolic pressure was 35 mmHg. The pulmonary flow was slightly more than twice the systemic flow.

4. Why should you search for a continuous murmur in the arms, legs, or abdomen in any patient in congestive failure of obscure etiology?

  ANS: A search must be made for an arteriovenous fistula, congenital or traumatic. If such a fistula is large (1 cm or more in diameter), signs and symptoms of failure may occur over a period of years.

5. What is the most common cause of a continuous murmur?

    ANS: **Persistent ductus arteriosus**, usually called patent ductus arteriosus or PDA. (All ducti are patent, otherwise it would be a ligamentum arteriosum.)

PDA Murmur
Shape and Duration

1. What are some of the other names for the continuous murmur of a PDA when it is truly continuous?

    ANS: A machinery or a Gibson murmur.

2. Why is a PDA murmur continuous?

    ANS: Because there is a continuous aortic-pulmonary pressure gradient throughout both systole and diastole (if the pulmonary artery pressure is not far from normal).

3. When is the continuous murmur of PDA not "machinery" in quality or duration?

    ANS: When it is not truly continuous, i.e., when it begins slightly after the S_1, crescendos to the S_2, and ends after a short decrescendo in early or mid-diastole.

    Note: About half of the PDA murmurs in children are not truly continuous, and many are only pansystolic, exactly mimicking a VSD murmur. This is because with the pulmonary vasoconstriction secondary to a large shunt, there is often a moderate degree of pulmonary hypertension, which decreases the aortic–pulmonary artery gradient more in diastole than in systole. In any child with a VSD type of pansystolic murmur a bounding pulse should make you strongly suspect a PDA.

4. Where in systole does the typical PDA murmur reach its maximum intensity?

    ANS: It is crescendo to a peak at or slightly before the S_2, and then is decrescendo to beyond the S_2.

Loudness and Site

1. Where is a PDA murmur heard (a) loudest and (b) next loudest?

    ANS: a. Loudest in the second left interspace.
         b. Next loudest in the first left interspace.

2. What is the significance of finding the next loudest site of a continuous murmur in the third left interspace?

    ANS: The diagnosis is not a PDA but some other cause of the continuous murmur, such as an aortic-pulmonary septal defect or a coronary artery communicating with either the coronary vein, right atrium, RV, or pulmonary artery.

Other Auscultatory Signs of PDA

1. What auscultatory signs of the increased flow through the mitral valve and large volume load on the LV may be heard in patients with a PDA?

   ANS: There may be an S_3 and/or a mitral diastolic flow murmur and the S_2 split may be paradoxical.

2. What are the multiple clicks or crackles heard at the end of systole and the beginning of diastole called? Their significance?

   ANS: Eddy sounds. They signify a large flow ductus [11].

PDA with High Pulmonary Artery Pressure

1. What causes differential cyanosis and clubbing (the feet cyanosed and clubbed, with the hand and face normal) in a PDA Eisenmenger situation, and why may the left hand be more cyanotic and clubbed than the right hand?

   ANS: With pulmonary hypertension, unsaturated blood flows through a ductus from the pulmonary artery to the aorta. The ductus often joins the pulmonary artery to the aorta just beyond the left subclavian artery. Unsaturated pulmonary artery blood will then pass beyond the left subclavian artery, and both hands will be less clubbed and cyanotic than the feet. If, however, the ductus is at the junction of the aorta and the left subclavian artery, the left hand will be as cyanotic and clubbed as the feet.

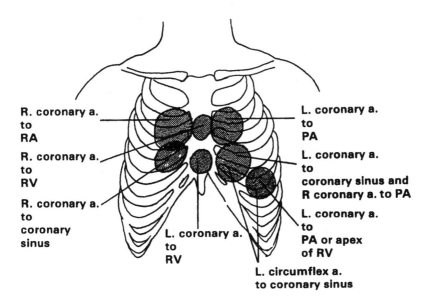

Coronary artery fistulas will often give a clue to their site of drainage by the site of the loudest murmur.

2. When will a right-to-left shunt (reversed ductus flow due to pulmonary hyper-tension) produce a murmur?

ANS: It is a general rule that right-to-left shunts do not produce murmurs.

The Venous Hum

1. Where is the venous hum best heard?

ANS: Just above the clavicle, either medial to the sternocleidomastoid muscle or between its insertions. A venous hum is more likely to be heard on the right side because the right jugular is larger than the left, since it must carry about two-thirds of the intracranial venous drainage.

2. What does a venous hum sound like?

ANS: Sometimes like a continuous roar; at other times like "the sound of the sea" heard by putting a seashell to the ear; and sometimes as a whining sound. The diastolic component is often higher-pitched and louder than the systolic. Probably the only quality that is never present is that of an actual hum!

3. What causes the venous hum?

ANS: Two theories have been proposed.

  a. Turbulence caused by a confluence of flow through the internal jugular and subclavian veins as they pour into the superior vena cave.

  b. Anterior angulation of the internal jugular vein by the transverse process of the atlas [12]. (This angulation and also the murmur can be shown to increase by turning the head away from the side of the hum.)

4. How can you elicit a venous hum if you cannot hear it by merely placing the stethoscope on the neck?

ANS: a. Ask the patient to sit up with his or her feet on the bed to bring maximum blood volume to the heart from both the lower body and head.

  b. Apply the small bell lightly to the right side of the neck, as closely as possible to the clavicle and anterior border of the sternocleidomastoid muscle or between its insertions. Too much pressure will eliminate the hum.

  c. Turn the patient's head away maximally and raise the chin as high as possible.

Note: The hum is often augmented by deep inspiration.

  d. When a continuous roar or whine is heard, test for the presence of a hum by applying moderate pressure with the fingers a few inches above the stethoscope. A venous hum will disappear with moderate pressure on the internal jugular vein.

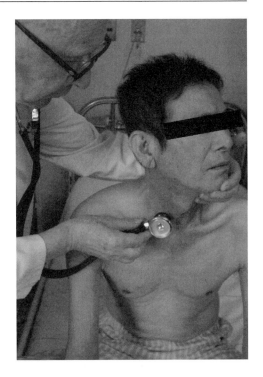

A small bell is invaluable in enabling you to apply airtight light pressure anterior to the sternomastoid muscle.

5. What is the significance of a venous hum that can be elicited without head-turning?

   ANS: It suggests that the **circulation time** is at least normal and may even be faster than normal. The unelicited venous hum is of most help in confirming the presence of hyperthyroidism in the young and in suggesting the diagnosis of apathetic hyperthyroidism in the elderly, i.e., hyperthyroidism with no apparent symptoms or signs of thyrotoxicosis and often with atrial fibrillation. The nonelicited venous hum is also common in patients with severe uremia with a low hematocrit as well as in pregnant women.

   Note: Although a venous hum should always be expected if you are diagnosing hyperthyroidism, the hum may disappear if the patient goes into enough heart failure to slow venous flow.

6. What are the methods of eliminating the venous hum besides applying pressure above or with the stethoscope?

   ANS: a. Turn the patient's head toward the side of the hum.
         b. Decrease venous return from the jugular veins by placing the patient in a supine position.

Note: Some hyperthyroid patients have a faint, high-frequency, continuous murmur, heard clearly over the thyroid after the venous hum has been eliminated by pressure over the jugular.

7. When does a venous hum mimic (a) PDA or (b) AR?

ANS: a. In some children the venous hum is transmitted downward to the upper chest, and since it sounds like a continuous murmur, it has been mistaken for the murmur of a PDA.

b. When only the diastolic component is transmitted downward and it is high-pitched.

Other Causes of Continuous Murmurs

1. What is meant by a pulmonary arteriovenous fistula?

ANS: This is a right-to-left shunt from pulmonary artery to pulmonary vein. It is usually congenital.

2. By inspection alone, what clues indicate that the continuous murmur is due to a pulmonary arteriovenous fistula.

ANS: Cyanosis, clubbing, and telangiectasia on the skin or mucous membranes.

3. What should you suspect as a cause of a continuous murmur that is heard bilaterally in a patient with cyanosis and a roentgenogram that suggests no pulmonary artery at all?

ANS: Bronchopulmonary anastamoses, i.e., large bronchial arteries supplying the lungs in a patient with:

a. A persistent truncus arteriosus (one large aorta-like vessel coming off both ventricles by straddling a VSD) with small pulmonary arteries, or

b. A solitary arterial trunk with pulmonary atresia.

4. What causes the continuous murmur of **coarctation**?

ANS: Although the systolic and diastolic pressure gradient across a severe coarctation has been shown by intra-aortic phonocardiography to produce a continuous murmur, collateral intercostal vessel flow is probably the most likely cause of a continuous murmur heard in coarctation. In mild or moderate coarctation, there is only a systolic murmur over the area of actual coarctation.

The Mammary Souffle

1. What is the cause of the mammary souffle?

ANS: It is an arterial murmur due to a large flow of blood into the breast during pregnancy and lactation in a minority of pregnant women.

Note: Firm pressure with the stethoscope can abolish the murmur. Palpable arterial pulsations in the relevant intercostal spaces are present in most cases.

2. What is the usual site and loudness of the mammary souffle?

ANS: It is usually heard along the left sternal border, and it is rarely more than grade 4/6.

Note: a. It may disappear when the patient sits up.
b. Although it usually begins in the second or third trimester, it may not begin until the first postpartum week and usually lasts from several weeks to 2 months postpartum.

3. What is characteristic of the timing of the mammary souffle?

ANS: There is a delay between the S_1 and the murmur, which often spills over the S_2 into early diastole. Therefore, it must be distinguished from other causes of continuous murmurs. It may be systolic, to-and-fro, or continuous. It is more common on the left than on the right.

Note: The gap between the S_1 and the onset of the murmur is due to the interval required for the blood ejected from the LV to arrive at the artery of origin.

REFERENCES

1. Agarwal, A. K. A new observation on papillary muscle dysfunction. *Chest* 82:130, 1982.
2. Fulkerson, P. K., et al. Calcification of the mitral annulus: Etiology, clinical associations complications and therapy. *Am. J. Med.* 66:967,1979.
3. Heikkila, J. Mitral incompetence complicating acute myocardial infarction. *Br. Heart J.* 29:162, 1967.
4. Auger, P., and Wigle, E. D. Sudden, severe mitral insufficiency. *Can. Med. Assoc. J.* 96:1493, 1967.
5. Dock, W. Production mode of systolic clicks due to mitral cusp prolapse. *Arch. Intern. Med.* 132:118, 1973.
6. Fujii, J., et al. Echocardiographic and phonocardiographic study on the genesis of the musical murmur. *J. Cardiogr.* 6:385, 1976.
7. Rivero-Carvallo, J. M. Signo para el diagnostico de las insuffiencias tricuspidias. *Arch. Inst. Cardiol. Mexico* 16:531, 1946.
8. Gooch, A. S., Cha, S. D., and Maranhao V. Tale use of the hepatic pressure maneuver to identify the murmur of tricuspid regurgitation. *Clin. Cardiol.* 6:277, 1983.
9. Yanagihara, K., et al. Phonocardiographic features of anomalous left coronary artery originating from the pulmonary artery: Report of two cases. *J. Cardiogr.* 8:147, 1978.

10. Haze, K., et al. Interventricular septal perforation secondary to acute myocardial infarction: Phonocardiographie appraisal of thirteen cases. *Cardiovasc. Sound Bull.* 5:593, 1975.
11. Hubbard, T. F., and Neis, D. D. The sounds at the base of the heart in cases of patent ductus arteriosus. *Am. Heart J.* 59:807, 1960.
12. Cutforth, R., Wiseman, J., and Sutherland, R. D. The genesis of the cervical venous hum. *Am. Heart J.* 80:488, 1970.

15 Diastolic Murmurs

DIASTOLIC ATRIOVENTRICULAR VALVE MURMURS ————

Mitral Stenosis Murmurs

Timing and Shape

1. When in the cycle does the diastolic murmur of mitral stenosis (MS) begin? How does it relate to the S_2?

   ANS: It begins just after the opening snap (OS). This means that there must be a pause between the A_2 and the diastolic murmur, a pause due to **isovolumic relaxation** of the left ventricle (LV). Because of the pause that usually occurs after the S_2, the MS murmur may be called an early delayed diastolic murmur.

2. What is the typical shape of the diastolic murmur of MS on auscultation? Why?

   ANS: After a very short crescendo, there is a decrescendo rumble that ends with a late crescendo to the M_1. The decrescendo reflects the decrescendo gradient and flow between the left atrium and the LV. The late crescendo has a more complicated explanation (see following section).

The Crescendo Murmur to the M_1 in Mitral Stenosis (The "Presystolic" Murmur)

1. What is the appearance or shape of a murmur that is produced by atrial contraction forcing blood through a stenotic mitral valve?

   ANS: It should follow the curve of atrial pressure rise and fall, i.e., it should be crescendo–decrescendo.

2. What is the actual shape of the diastolic murmur produced by atrial contraction at the end of diastole in MS?

   ANS: It is crescendo to the first sound. This murmur is often called "presystolic."

3. Does the presystolic crescendo murmur of MS extend to the M_1?

   ANS: Yes.

Boldface type indicates that the term is explained in the glossary.

243

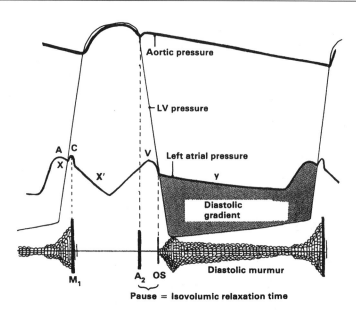

There should be no mitral murmurs between the A_2 and the OS, because this is isovolumic relaxation time. Note the slow Y descent of the left atrium due to the difficulty in emptying the left atrium through the stenotic valve. This accounts for the pressure gradient and murmur, both of which are decrescendo except for the very beginning and end.

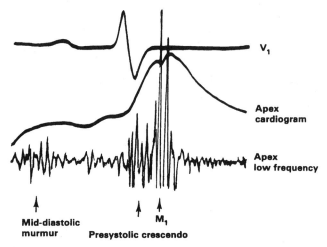

The "preystolic" murmur in this 45-year-old woman with moderately severe MS begins with the onset of ventricular contraction, as shown by the simultaneous apex cardiogram tracing taken at very fast paper speed. However, blood is still flowing from the left atrium to the LV until mitral valve closure (M_1). Therefore, cardiologists prefer to consider this period as part of diastole.

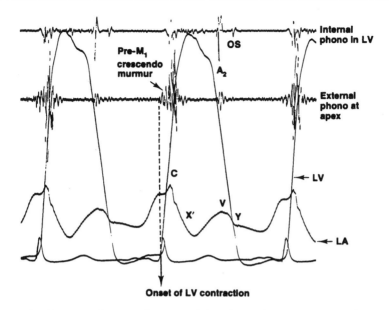

Onset of LV contraction

These simultaneous phonocardiograms, left atrial und LV pressure tracings were taken with catheter-tip micromanonieter pressure transducers to eliminate any time delays due to tubing. Note that the "presystolic" crescendo of the MS murmur occurs during ventricular systole. This is from a 43-year-old man, mildly symptomatic, with severe MS, but only a small amount of calcium in his mitral valve. His left atrial A wave was 32 mmHg, but his cardiac index was 2.7, which is low-normal. He had a grade 3/6 diastolic rumble at the apex, of which only the presystolic component is seen well in these phonocarcdiograms.

4. What may we call the time between ventricular contraction and closure of the mitral valve or M_1?

   ANS: The preisovolumic contraction period.

   Note: This period is prolonged in MS because both the high left atrial pressure and the stiffness of the mitral valve have to be overcome before the mitral valve can be closed.

5. If the presystolic crescendo murmur actually occurs during LV contraction, i.e., during the preisovolumic LV contraction period, is it really presystolic?

   ANS: If systole is defined as beginning with ventricular contraction (physiologists' systole), then only the first part of the murmur in sinus rhythm is presystolic because it begins at the time of peak atrial contraction before the ventricle contracts. Most of the murmur, however, is actually an early systolic murmur because it occurs during the preisovolumic contraction period of LV contraction. This is apparent from the observation that most of the crescendo murmur to the M_1 occurs after the onset of the QRS. However, because the auscultator's systole begins with the S_1, it is not necessary to change the traditional terminology of presyscolic murmur. By a presystolic murmur, then, the auscultator means "immediately before the first heart sound."

6. What is the probable cause of the presystolic crescendo?

    ANS: As the mitral valve orifice is being reduced by LV contraction the velocity of forward flow is increasing as long as the pressure is higher in the left atrium than in the LV [1].

7. Is atrial contraction required to produce the presystolic crescendo murmur?

    ANS: No. In atrial fibrillation the late crescendo occurs but only during short diastoles, because only during short diastoles is the left atrial pressure high enough to maintain high-velocity flow during preisovolumic ventricular contraction. This also explains why sinus rhythm and atrial contraction helps to produce the pre-M_1 crescendo. Atrial contraction can elevate left atrial pressure sufficiently to create the necessary increased velocity of forward flow as the mitral valve orifice is being reduced by ventricular contraction.

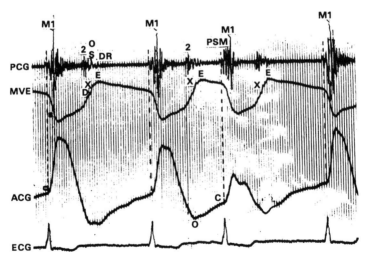

Presystolic murmur in a patient with mitral stenosis and atrial fibrillation. The best presystolic crescendo to the M_1, occurring at the end of a short diastole begins with the start of mitral valve closure on the mitral valve "gated" echocardiogram (MVE) and with the start of LV contraction, point C of the apex cardiogram (ACG). The presystolic murmur occurs during preisovolumic LV contraction. (From P. Toutouzas et al. Mechanism of diastolic rumble and presystolic murmur in mitral stenosis. *Br. Heart J.* 36:1096, 1974.)

Pitch and Quality

1. Is the MS diastolic murmur high or low in pitch? Why?

   ANS: Low, because a murmur that is produced more by flow than by **gradient** produces mostly low frequencies. The gradient across the mitral valve in diastole is relatively low as gradients go, no matter how severe the stenosis is; i.e. even in severe MS, the maximum diastolic gradient is about 30 mmHg at the beginning of diastole and about 10 mmHg at the end. In aortic or pulmonary stenosis peak systolic gradients with moderate to severe obstructions during systole are at least 50 mmHg and may exceed 100 mmHg.

2. What are some of the descriptions of the MS diastolic murmur that help to symbolize the low frequencies?

   ANS: Rumbling, like distant thunder, like a ball rolling down a bowling alley, and blubbering (Austin Flint used this word in 1884).

   Note: The early rumble followed by a late crescendo to a loud M_1 may be likened to the growl (rumble) and bark (late crescendo) of a dog.

Factors That Increase the Loudness of Mitral Stenosis Murmurs

1. How can you bring out a mitral diastolic murmur that is almost inaudible?

   ANS: a. Bring the LV closer to the stethoscope by turning the patient to the **left lateral decubitus position**. Listen during end-expiration over the site where your finger feels the apex beat because soft MS murmurs are often extremely localized precisely over the apex beat.

   b. Use very light pressure with the largest bell available that will allow a good air seal. Firm pressure can completely obliterate the low frequencies of a faint rumble.

   c. Increase the flow across the mitral valve.

2. How can you increase the flow across the mitral valve?

   ANS a. Have the patient cough a few times, or listen after a **Valsalva** strain during the release phase. In the post-Valsalva release phase, the obstructed vena caval venous flow floods the lungs and pours into the left atrium a few seconds later. There is a more pronounced post-Valsalva rise of pressure in the left atrium in MS than in the normal heart [2].

   b. If the heart rate is fast, listen after digitalis or a beta or calcium blocker has slowed the rate and increased the volume of diastolic flow into the LV. (Digitalis may also increase the force of LV expansion or "suction.")

c. Listen when the patient is squatting or during a handgrip maneuver. Cardiac output is increased for a few beats immediately upon squatting. During handgrip the mitral diastolic gradient has been shown to increase as a result of both the increase in cardiac output and the increase in heart rate [3].

d. Ask the patient to exercise. (Merely turning the patient to the left lateral decubitus position may be sufficient, and you should listen immediately, before the effect of the exertion is lost.) The maximum effective duration for the supine straight leg-raising exercise beyond which there is probably not much more increase in cardiac output is, at the most, 3 min, i.e., physiologists consider 3 min of moderate exercise sufficient to reach a steady state. The more vigorous the exercise the longer it takes to reach a steady state.

e. Administer amyl nitrite. (See p. 224 for an explanation of how amyl nitrite increases venous return and cardiac output.)

Factors that Make the Mitral Stenosis Murmur Softer

1. What can make MS diastolic murmurs soft besides mild MS, obesity, or emphysema?

    ANS: a. Low flow.

    b. A large right ventricle (RV) pushing the LV posteriorly. The RV is an anterior chamber, and if it enlarges, as it often does in MS, it pushes the LV away from the anterior chest wall.

2. What besides the mitral obstruction itself can cause a low flow in MS?

    ANS: a. Severe pulmonary hypertension. This causes an additional obstruction to flow for which RV hypertrophy and a rise in RV pressure do not compensate completely.

    b. Other valves causing obstruction, i.e., tricuspid or aortic stenosis.

    c. A **cardiomyopathy**, usually on either a rheumatic or coronary basis.

    d. Atrial fibrillation. Atrial fibrillation often causes too fast a ventricular rate for good diastolic flow through the mitral obstruction but even when the heart rates are slow, the loss of atrial contraction reduces flow. A well-placed atrial contraction can increase cardiac output by about 25% in significant MS.

Etiologies and Differential Diagnosis

1. What is the usual etiology of MS?

    ANS: Rheumatic fever which causes a chronic process of valvular fibrosis, fusion, and calcification, together with shortened, thickened chordae tendineae.

    Note: The normal valve orifice measures $4-6$ cm^2. It must be reduced to about 2.5 cm^2 to elevate left atrial pressure significantly enough to produce symptoms. Severe, tight stenosis occurs at 1 cm^2.

2. What are the most common imitators of the MS diastolic murmur despite no significant diastolic gradient across the mitral valve?

    ANS: a. A diastolic flow murmur due to excessive flow across the mitral valve, as in severe mitral regurgitation (MR).

    b. The Austin Flint murmur.

3. What auscultatory clues indicate that a mitral diastolic rumble may not be due to true MS?

    ANS: MS is not likely if

    a. An S_3 precedes a short murmur. Only rarely does a true S_3 precede any MS murmur, but if it does, the murmur will be long and loud.

    b. There is no good presystolic crescendo.

    c. There is no loud S_1 or opening snap.

    d. It varies in loudness and position from beat to beat and from one position to another. This is characteristic of a left atrial myxoma. (May be grade 4/6.)

    Note: The finding of a low-frequency diastolic rumble across a St. Jude Medical or Byork-Shiley prosthesis in the mitral position, although occasionally a normal finding, should prompt careful evaluation.

The Austin Flint Murmur Versus the Mitral Stenosis Murmur

1. What is the Austin Flint murmur [4]?

    ANS: It is an apical diastolic rumble imitating the murmur of organic MS but is due to an aortic regurgitation (AR) stream that prevents the mitral valve from opening fully.

2. What is the most plausible theory explaining the mechanical cause of the Austin Flint murmur?

    ANS: The AR stream may impinge on the undersurface of the anterior leaflet of the mitral valve and push it up, creating a relative MS. Support for this theory is found in the following:

    a. A yellow plaque (jet lesion) occurs on the septal surface of the anterior mitral leaflet of some patients with the Austin Flint murmur [5].

    b. When an Austin Flint murmur is present, the amplitude of opening of the mitral anterior leaflet is reduced on echocardiograms.

    Note: Echocardiograms often show fluttering of the anterior mitral leaflet in patients with Austin Flint murmurs. This was once thought to be the cause of the murmur, but some patients with the fluttering leaflets have no Austin Flint murmur, and some with the Austin Flint murmur have no flutter.

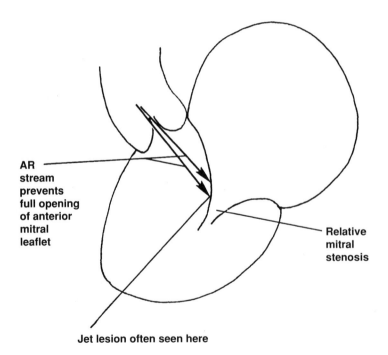

Jet lesion often seen here

The aortic regurgitant (AR) stream holds the anterior leaflet up into a semiclosed position. This accounts for the mitral diastolic rumble mimicking mitral stenosis and for the attenuated opening snap in patients with both mitral stenosis und aortic regurgitation.

3. What suggests that the apical diastolic murmur in severe AR is at least sometimes due to transmission of the low-frequency components of the AR murmur
   to the apex?

   ANS: It sometimes starts with the S_2, i.e., before the mitral valve has had a
         chance to open, and persists at end of diastole even when mitral
         inflow has ceased (by Doppler) when LV pressure has exceeded left
         atrial pressure.

4. Is there a presystolic crescendo in the Austin Flint murmur?

   ANS   Rarely. The presystolic accentuation of the Austin Flint murmur even
         when present is often a subtle finding and does not have a marked cre-
         scendo to the S_1.

   Note: Austin Flint called the murmur "presystolic." But he also wrote that
            the classical pandiastolic murmur of pure mitral stenosis was also
            "presystolic"

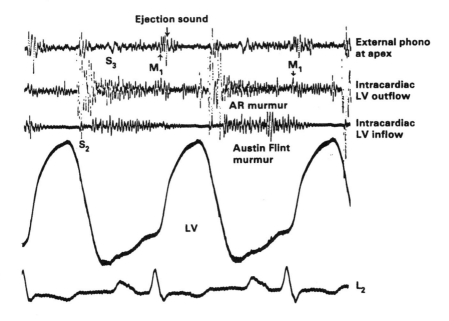

Phonocardiograms and LV pressure tracing from a 45-year-old man with marked
orthopnea who had an Austin Flint murmur due to severe AR resulting from a
previous infective endocarditis. Note that the diastolic rumble at the apex begins
even before the S_3 was recorded externally. Note also the absence of a presystolic
crescendo and the soft M_1.

5. How can you differentiate an Austin Flint murmur from the murmur of MS by auscultation?

    ANS: a. If there is no OS, the chances that MS is present are diminished. But remember that AR can attenuate or eliminate an OS.

              b. If there is no obvious presystolic crescendo to the S_1, it is more likely to be an Austin Flint murmur.

              c. Amyl nitrite will produce a louder MS murmur after about 20 s, whereas an Austin Flint murmur immediately becomes softer or even disappears. The reason for this is that in AR there are two outlets for aortic blood during diastole, one outlet backward into the LV, the other forward into the peripheral arteries. Amyl nitrite lowers peripheral resistance, thus increasing the peripheral run-off, and therefore decreasing the amount of AR.

Mitral Diastolic Flow Murmurs (Inflow Murmurs)

1. What is meant by a mitral diastolic inflow murmur?

    ANS: This murmur is a low-pitched rumble heard over the apex area that is produced by a relative or functional MS, i.e., by an excessive flow through a normal mitral valve.

2. List some common causes of excessive flow through a mitral valve that can produce a diastolic flow murmur besides severe MR and hyperkinetic states such as thyrotoxicosis.

    ANS: a. The very slow ventricular rate of congenital complete **atrioventricular** (AV) **block**.

              b. A large left-to-right shunt, e.g., a **persistent ductus arteriosus** or VSD.

3. In which way does a mitral diastolic flow murmur differ from the murmur of MS?

    ANS: A flow murmur usually starts with an S_3, is short, and has no late diastolic or presystolic component.

4. Why does the diastolic flow murmur not start exactly with the onset of opening of the mitral valve?

    ANS: The fully open mitral valve makes too large an orifice for a murmur to be produced. Echocardiograms have shown that immediately after the initial opening movement of the mitral valve, the valve moves rapidly into a semiclosed position, probably as a result of eddy currents. The murmur is thus probably due to the increasing velocity of flow as a result of a dynamically narrowing mitral orifice, much like the effect of narrowing the nozzle of a hose.

5. What is meant by a Carey Coombs murmur?

ANS: It is the diastolic inflow murmur usually ushered in by an S_3, heard in subjects with cardiomegaly and MR due to acute rheumatic fever [6].

TRICUSPID DIASTOLIC FLOW MURMURS

1. What is the site of the tricuspid inflow murmur?

ANS: Anywhere over the RV area. This includes all the lower right and left parasternal area as well as the epigastrium. When the RV is very large, the entire left lower chest area can also become the RV area.

2. List the common causes of increased diastolic flow through the tricuspid valve.

ANS: a. Shunt flows, e.g., **atrial septal defect** (ASD) and **anomalous pulmonary venous connection** or drainage into a right atrium.
b. Tricuspid regurgitation (TR).

TRICUSPID STENOSIS (TS) DIASTOLIC MURMURS

1. Where is the TS murmur heard on the chest wall?

ANS: In the same place as the tricuspid inflow murmur, i.e., the RV area.

2. How does the TS murmur differ from the MS murmur?

ANS: a. In sinus rhythm it is only a presystolic murmur but has no presystolic crescendo to the S_1, i.e., the TS presystolic murmur is nearly always a short crescendo–decrescendo murmur and therefore sounds like an S_4 murmur. Only if atrial fibrillation is present is there only a delayed early diastolic murmur.
b. It always increases with inspiration, often markedly, whereas the MS murmur characteristically decreases with inspiration.
c. The MS murmur is louder in the left lateral decubitus position. The TS murmur is accentuated in the right lateral decubitus position.
d. The MS murmur is usually predominantly low-pitched and rumbling; the TS presystolic murmur is often scratchy. It is higher pitched and more superficial than the MS murmur.

3. What is the significance of a TS murmur in the absence of MS?

ANS: Rheumatic TS is probably never present without MS even though on rare occasions the TS may be the dominant lesion. Therefore if no MS can be diagnosed, a presystolic murmur at the left sternal border should make you suspect either a right atrial myxoma or an ASD.

4. Does the TS murmur increase with held inspiration?

   ANS: It increases both during moving inspiration and during inspiratory apnea.

   Note: Look for "suffusion sign": on lying flat, the face becomes cyanotic and the scalp veins become dilated.

DIASTOLIC SEMILUNAR VALVE MURMURS

Aortic Regurgitation Murmurs

Causes of Aortic Regurgitation

1. What are the most common causes of severe AR (a) in the child, and (b) in the adult?

   ANS: a. In the young child, a VSD with aortic valve prolapse may be the most common cause of severe AR.

         b. In the adult, rheumatic heart disease, endocarditis, or paraprosthetic valve leaks are probably equally common as causes of severe AR.

2. What is the most common cause of mild AR in the adult? Why?

   ANS: Severe hypertension. In one series of severely hypertensive patients, 60% had AR [7]. When the diastolic pressure is reduced below 115 mmHg, the AR may disappear. Two causes have been suggested: (a) dilatation of the aortic annulus and (b) high pressure above a bicuspid or fenestrated aortic valve.

   Note: a. Bicuspid aortic valves occur in about 2% of males and 1% of females.

         b. Fenestrations are common in both aortic and pulmonary valves.

         c. The aortic annulus is not significantly dilated at systolic pressures below 170, or diastolic-pressures below 105.

3. List some rare causes of AR (a) with arthritis and (b) without arthritis.

   ANS: a. With arthritis:

             (1) Ankylosing spondylitis.
             (2) Reiter's syndrome. In about 5% with this syndrome, AR may be found from 1 to 20 years after diagnosis.
             (3) Rheumatoid or psoriatic arthritis.

         b. Without arthritis:

             (1) Syphilis (leutic aortitis).
             (2) Osteogenesis imperfecta. The AR here is due to dilatation of the aortic root.
             (3) Dissecting aneurysm of the ascending aorta.
             (4) Rupture of a **sinus of Valsalva**.
             (5) The **Marfan syndrome**. The AR is due to dilatation of the aortic root and myxomatous degeneration of the cusps.

Note: Although both males and females with the Marfan syndrome may have MR, only males (usually under age 40) develop AR. Although myxomatous transformation of the aortic valve is characteristic of the Marfan syndrome, it can occur without this syndrome; when it does, it can result in rupture of an aortic cusp.

4. What should make you suspect by auscultation that a bicuspid aortic valve is the cause of the AR?

    ANS: Mild AR plus an ejection click followed by an early ejection murmur that is loudest in the second right interspace. The A_2 may also be loud and snapping.

Timing and Shape

1. When in the cycle does the AR murmur begin, and what is its shape?

    ANS: It begins with the aortic component of the second sound (A_2). In general, it is decrescendo.

    Note: There is often a very early and very short crescendo–decrescendo to the murmur if the AR is not more than moderate.

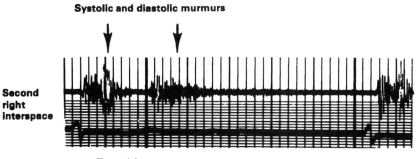

This murmur was due to mild syphilitic AR. It was loudest at the second and third right interspaces. Note the slight early crescendo–decrescendo. A systolic murmur due to blood going in one direction, together with a diastolic murmur due to blood going in the opposite direction, is called a to-and-fro murmur.

2. What is the auscultatory effect on the short and early crescendo–decrescendo?

    ANS: The murmur appears to start after a short silent period following the A_2. The background rhythm effect is as follows:

    1——2–HAaaaaa–1——2–HAaaaaa

Quality and Loudness

1. What is the dominant frequency or pitch of the usual AR murmur? Why?

   ANS: The dominant frequency is high. If the AR is mild, then the murmur will be due more to a large gradient than to flow, and the murmur will therefore be purely high-pitched and blowing. If the AR is moderate, the murmur will be due to a greater flow as well as to a high-velocity jet, and it will have mixed frequencies but still be dominantly high. If the AR is severe, the murmur may be very rough due to an excess of low and medium frequencies.

   Note: Although the more low frequencies there are the more severe the AR, the reverse is not necessarily true, i.e., a pure high-frequency murmur may be present with moderately severe AR. Presumably the low-frequency components are transmitted to areas not accessible to the stethoscope.

2. How can you best imitate by voice the sound of a typical mild AR murmur, i.e., a purely high-pitched murmur?

   ANS: In Mexico this has been called an "aspirative" AR murmur and is imitated by breathing in noisily through the mouth. If you breathe out quickly with the mouth open or whisper "ah," you can easily imitate the classic AR murmur.

   Note: Because it sounds so much like a breath sound, the patient should hold his or her breath in expiration to allow you to perceive this murmur better.

3. How can you increase the loudness of the very soft AR murmur?

   ANS: a. The standard method is to get the stethoscope closer to the heart by having the patient sit up and lean forward. Then press hard with the stethoscope diaphragm over the sternum or left sternal border during held expiration. Another method, not widely known, is to do the same but with the patient in the left lateral decubitus position.

   b. You can increase peripheral resistance. To do this:

   (1) Ask the patient to squat and auscultate the patient's chest immediately. The increase in venous return for a few beats will also help increase the murmur; and/or

   (2) Have the patient do isometric exercise by means of a handgrip. The elevation of systolic blood pressure after 3 min of 33% maximum handgrip pressure is greater in patients with AR than in normal subjects.

   (3) Administer a vasopressor drug.

   Note: A soft AR murmur (or MR murmur) may disappear in pregnancy, owing to the fall in resistance.

4. What is the significance of a musical AR vibratory or "dove-coo" AR murmur?

   ANS: Musical aortic diastolic murmurs often occur in patients with a perfo-
   rated leaflet, as in infective endocarditis, everted leaflets (often luetic), or
   rupture of an aortic **sinus of Valsalva**. Ruptures of leaflets are usually
   secondary to myxomatous transformation or infective endocarditis.

L. lower sternal border   High frequency

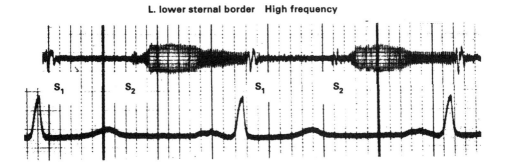

Luetic AR was suspected as the cause of this aortic diastolic murmur. Note the regular
vibrations seen in all phonocardiograms of musical murmurs.

Site of AR Murmurs

1. Where, as a rule, is the AR murmur best heard?

   ANS: Just to the left of the sternum at the level of the third or fourth intercostal space.

2. When is the AR murmur best heard to the *right* of the sternum?

   ANS: In the presence of marked poststenotic dilatation of the aorta (when AS
   is also present) or when marked atherosclerotic tortuosity pushes the
   ascending aorta anteriorly and to the right. It is best heard in the *fourth*
   right interspace only if it is due to nonrheumatic conditions that cause
   the regurgitant stream to flow in peculiar directions; e.g., when it is
   secondary to infective endocarditis, an aortic aneurysm, a prolapsed
   aortic valve, or a rupture of a **sinus of Valsalva**.

3. What other unusual murmur radiations are occasionally found in AR?

   ANS: The murmur may be even louder in the high mid-left thorax, at the
   apex, or in the mid-axillary line than at the sternal edge. This has been
   called the Cole-Cecil murmur [8]. The cause for these unusual radiations is unknown. Occasionally the murmur may even be heard *only* in
   the axillary area or at the apex.

Sudden, Severe Aortic Regurgitation

1. What are the most likely causes of sudden severe AR?

    ANS: (a) **Infective endocarditis**, and

    (b) rupture of an aneurysm of a **sinus of Valsalva**.

2. How are the heart sounds and diastolic murmurs affected by sudden severe AR?

    ANS: The S_1 is soft or absent and there may be a loud S_3-like sound in mid-diastole due to closure of the mitral valve. The diastolic murmur tends to be relatively short and soft.

    Note: a. In some cases of acute severe AR, the blood pressure may be average, i.e., in the range of 115/75 instead of the usual high systolic and low diastolic of chronic severe AR.

    b. The tachycardia of sudden, severe AR often causes diastole to equal, or even be shorter than, systole, so that it is difficult to tell systole from diastole by auscultation. This occurs because ejection is prolonged by the severe LV volume overload, and the diastolic period may be further shortened by tachycardia. Carotid or apical palpation during auscultation is mandatory to avoid confusing systole with diastole.

PULMONARY REGURGITATION MURMURS

Murmurs with High Pressure in the Pulmonary Artery (Graham Steell Murmur)

1. How high does the pulmonary artery pressure have to be to produce a pulmonary regurgitation (PR) murmur?

    ANS: It is usually at nearly systemic levels. Pulmonary regurgitation murmurs are rarely present with pulmonary artery pressures of below 80 mmHg systolic unless the main pulmonary artery is markedly dilated.

    Note: A Graham Steell murmur is a PR murmur that is secondary to pulmonary hypertension.

2. How does the Graham Steell murmur differ from the AR murmur?

    ANS: It may not differ, i.e., both are dominantly high-pitched and may be from grade 1 to 6. The Graham Steell murmur, however, often increases with inspiration and also increases with amyl nitrate, while AR decreases.

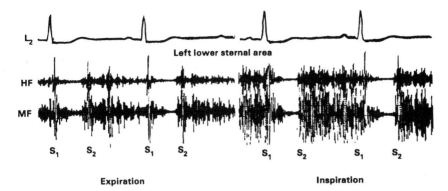

These phonocardiograms are from a patient with a PDA whose pulmonary artery pressure was 145 mmHg, with an aortic pressure about the same. This loud diastolic murmur (Graham Steell murmur) increased markedly on inspiration. A soft Graham Steell murmur may not increase with inspiration.

PR Murmurs with Normal Pressures in the Pulmonary Artery (Primary PR)

1. What is the most common cause of a primary PR murmur, besides surgery on the pulmonary valve?

    ANS: Idiopathic dilatation of the pulmonary artery.

2. How do the shape, length, and pitch of a primary PR murmur differ from those of the Graham Steell murmur?

    ANS: In PR with *normal* pressures in the pulmonary artery, there is sometimes a slight delay after the P_2 before any murmur is heard. However, even if it starts with the P_2, the murmur tends to be short and rough, due to dominant medium and low frequencies. (See figure on p. 260.)

PERICARDIAL FRICTION RUBS

Pericarditis

1. What is the mechanism that causes friction rubs?

    ANS: It is usually assumed that the rub sounds are caused by the two roughened pericardial membranes (the visceral and parietal pericardia) sliding over each other. However, when the overlying pleura is also involved, perhaps the noises are caused by the pleura rubbing against the outer layer of pericardium. The rub then would be a pleuropericardial friction rub.

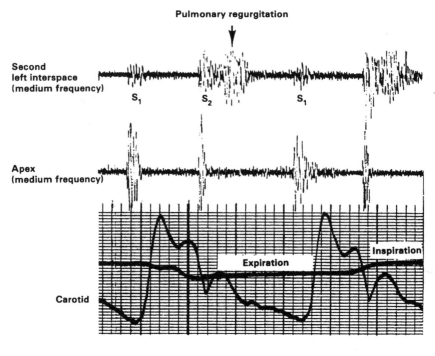

Primary PR

This murmur of primary PR in a teen-age boy was early diastolic and had many low and medium frequencies in it. It did not increase with inspiration at the second left interspace because too much air was interposed between heart and stethoscope in that area. The murmur was softer at the left lower sternal border, where, however, it did become louder with inspiration.

> *Note*: The three most common causes of generalized pericarditis are viral peri-carditis, disseminated lupus, and uremia.

2. What is the most common cause of a localized pericarditis?

   ANS: Acute myocardial infarction.

   Note: a. If there has been neither infarction nor trauma to the heart (includ-ing radiation to the chest), then consider a metastatic tumor involv-ing the heart.

   b. Inability to extend the neck is common in pericarditis. Patients may lie prone and flexed on their pillows.

How to Recognize a Pericardial Friction Rub

1. What adjectives and analogies have been used to describe the quality of friction rubs?

   ANS: They are usually described as crunching, scraping, creaking, grating, crackling, or scratching. They often sound like squeaky shoes or like two pieces of sandpaper rubbed against one another. Occasionally, however, they sound no different from any mixed-frequency murmur. They often sound surprisingly superficial, and increased stethoscope pressure sometimes seems to make them unexpectedly louder. They may sound as if they are halfway up the stethoscope tubing.

2. How many components are heard in most friction rubs?

   ANS: Three: one systolic and two diastolic.

3. At what time in diastole do the two diastolic rubs occur?

   ANS: a. In early diastole, near the end of early rapid expansion of the ventricle, at the time when an S_3 would occur.

   b. At the end of diastole, when atrial contraction produces sudden ventricular expansion. This is the moment when an S_4 would occur.

4. Where in systole may a systolic rub occur?

   ANS: Anywhere. It may replace the first or second heart sound or occur only in mid-systole.

5. If one major rub replaces the first heart sound (the commonest occurrence) and two rubs occur in diastole, what is the cadence of the friction rubs that is heard as a background rhythm?

   ANS: The cadence is the same as that of a quadruple rhythm due to a double gallop, i.e.,

   > "ch–DUP–sh–sh———ch–DUP–sh–sh
   >   1   2   1   2

   Note: Because the systolic rub may replace both the S_1 and the S_2, it is common to hear the rhythm as "CH–sh–sh———CH–sh–sh." When one of the diastolic rubs is absent, it is usually the S_3, i.e., an S_4 rub is the last to disappear, probably because the heart is maximally distended at the end of diastole, tending to bring the inflamed pericardial surfaces into contact.

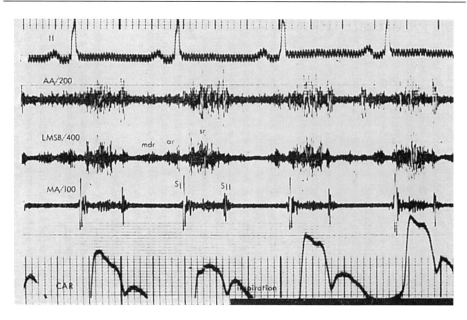

Triphasic pericardial friction rub. A rub is recorded during atrial systole (ar), ventricular systole (sr), and mid-diastole (mdr). (From Spodick, D. H.: Acoustic phenomena in pericardial disease. *Am. Heart J.* 81:114–124, 1971. Reprinted with permission).

6. Is the friction rub usually louder during inspiration or expiration? Why?

   ANS: In at least one-third of patients, it increases during inspiration [9]. This may be due to several possible causes:

   a. The downward pull of the diaphragm on the pericardium may draw the pericardium more tautly over the heart. The diaphragm is attached to the pericardium, and it is conceivable that a small amount of fluid between the visceral and parietal pericardia could be squeezed out by the tightening of the two layers with inspiration.

   b. It may be a pleuropericardial rub. Even when there is a pericardial effusion, there may still be a pericardial rub, and this may be accounted for either by the squeezing out of a small amount of fluid by inspiration or by the expanded lung pressing on the pericardium during inspiration. Therefore, in the presence of effusion the rub may only be heard with the patient supine in full inspiration.

7. Of the three major rub components, which one is almost always present? Which is the next most common component?

   ANS: The systolic component is almost always present. The atrial systolic component is next in frequency of occurrence, but rarely does an atrial systolic rub occur alone as the only rub sound. It almost always occurs together with at least a systolic rub.

Note: You can exaggerate a doubtful rub by having the patient lie on elbows and knees to promote apposition of the visceral and parietal pericardium. This is especially useful when only the systolic phase remains.

8. Where are most friction rubs best heard?

   ANS: Near the left sternal border, at about the third or fourth left interspace.

9. When is the friction rub transient?

   ANS: During the course of acute myocardial infarction, when it may last only a few hours.

   Note: In **postmyocardial infarction syndrome (Dressier's syndrome)**, it may last for weeks.

10. In what clinical setting, besides uremia, is a pericardial friction rub most likely?

    ANS: Immediately after open heart surgery.

    Note: Immediately postoperative, a crunchy noise at the apex synchronous with the heart beat in the left lateral decubitus position is Hamman's sign of air in the mediastinum.

REFERENCES

1. Criley, J. M., and Hermer, A. J. The crescendo presystolic murmur of mitral stenosis with atrial fibrillation. *N. Engl. J. Med.* 285:1284, 1971.
2. Bjork, V. O., and Malmstrom, G. Simultaneous left and right atrial pressure curves during Valsalva's experiment. *Am. Heart J.* 50:742, 1955.
3. Fisher, M. L., et al. Haemodynamic response to isometric exercise (handgrip) in patients with heart disease. *Br. Heart J.* 35:422, 1973.
4. Flint, A. *Disease of the Heart* (2nd ed.), Philadelphia: Henry C. Lea, 1870. pp. 206, 208.
5. Edwards, J. E., and Burchell, H. B. Endocardial and intimal lesions (jet impact). *Circulation* 18:946, 1958.
6. Coombs, C. F. Rheumatic myocardilis. *Quart. J. Med.* 2:26, 1908.
7. Luisada, A. A. The phonocardiogram in hypertension. *Chest* 58:598, 1970.
8. Cole, R., and Cecil, A. B. The axillary diastolic murmur in aortic insufficiency. *Bull. Johns Hopkins Hosp.* 19:353, 1908.
9. Spodick, D. H. Pericardial friction. *N. Engl. J. Med.* 278:1204, 1968.

16 Abdominal Murmurs

1. List the common causes of abdominal murmurs.

   ANS: a. Normal arterial and venous flow murmurs, usually heard only in young people.
   b. Stenosis of the aorta or of a renal, splenic, superior mesenteric, or iliac artery.
   c. Hepatic malignancies, alcoholic hepatitis, and portal-systemic vein anastomoses in portal hypertension.

NORMAL ABDOMINAL MURMURS

1. How common are abdominal murmurs in normal subjects?

   ANS: They occur in almost half of subjects under age 25 but in only about 5% of those over age 50. (Thus, an abdominal murmur in an older adult should probably be considered abnormal [1].)

2. Where are normal abdominal murmurs heard?

   ANS: Normal murmurs are heard in the epigastrium or over the inferior vena cave, where a venous hum is heard in about 5% of normal subjects [2].

   Note: a. In very thin patients, the murmur may radiate to the left lower sternal border of the chest and may be confused with a cardiac murmur.
   b. Most epigastric bruits are due to celiac artery stenosis.

ABNORMAL ABDOMINAL MURMURS

1. What is the pitch and timing of the stenosing renal vascular lesion murmur?

   ANS: It is high-pitched, sometimes to and fro with systolic accentuation, sometimes only a short systolic murmur, and sometimes continuous.

   Note: a. The kind of renal artery lesion that is most likely to have an arterial murmur is fibromuscular dysplasia.
   b. A continuous murmur means either an arteriovenous fistula of the portal system or renal artery stenosis.

    c. If a venous hum is present over the xiphoid region or umbilicus and is heard over the chest, suspect hepatic cirrhosis with portal systemic anastomoses (Cruveilhier-Baumgarten syndrome). Systolic accentuation occurs with inspiration or sitting up. Firm pressure at the site of a thrill may cause the murmur to disappear.

2. Where are the best sites for hearing renal vascular murmurs?

    ANS: Beneath the costal margin anteriorly, lateral to the aorta and lumbar spine. Renal artery stenosis murmurs are usually 2–4 in. lateral to the midepigastrium. Occasionally they are heard in the flanks over the kidneys.

    Note: An epigastric murmur is more likely to be due to celiac artery compression than to renal artery stenosis. Pulsations of the normal abdominal aorta do not extend below the umbilicus, and such a pulsation even in thin individuals suggests an aneurysm.

REFERENCES

1. Zoneraich, S., and Zoneraich O. Value of auscultation and phonoarteriography in detecting atherosclerotic involvement of the abdominal aorta and its branches. *Am. Heart J.* 83:620, 1972.
2. Rivin, A. U. Abdominal vascular sounds. *JAMA* 221:688. 1972.

Glossary

aneurysm Localized dilatation of either a blood vessel or a heart chamber. The most common cause of an arterial aneurysm is atherosclerosis. Anywhere in the aorta atrophy of the media (muscular layer) deep to an atherosclerotic plaque results in either a saccular or a fusiform (spindle-shaped) dilatation. The most common site is the abdomen distal to the renal arteries. Syphilis (lues) used to be the most common cause of thoracic aortic aneurysm, usually in the ascending aorta. When infection destroys a local area of any artery to cause a local dilatation, a mycotic aneurysm is said to have formed.

> **dissecting aneurysm** In the correct pronunciation the "diss" rhymes with "kiss." Localized aortic dilatation that results from separation of the layers of the aortic wall by hemorrhage into the media secondary to degeneration of the media (cystic medial necrosis). In some patients it may begin with an intimal tear. It usually dissects distally, but when it dissects proximally, it may involve the aortic valve and produce aortic regurgitation, or it may dissect into the pericardial space, producing a fatal tamponade.

> **ventricular aneurysm** A dilated segment of the left ventricle (LV). It is commonly caused by myocardial infarction. They vary in size from a few centimeters in diameter to a size one-half that of the LV. They rarely rupture but can cause heart failure. A thrombus often fills the aneurysm. It may bulge during systole (paradoxical motion or dyskinesis). A large area of damaged myocardium that fails to show any motion during systole is sometimes also called an aneurysm, although it is better simply to call this area akinetic or, if the movement is slight, hypokinetic.

anomalous pulmonary venous connection or drainage Drainage of one or more pulmonary veins, usually into the right atrium or superior or inferior vena cava. More rarely, a vein (or veins) from the left lung empties into the innominate vein, a left vertical vein, or the coronary sinus. The anomalous connection results in a left-to-right shunt with the same chambers overloaded as in atrial septal defect. In *total anomalous pulmonary venous return*, all of the pulmonary veins may enter any of the following: a left vertical vein, the innominate vein, the coronary sinus, the right atrium, the superior or inferior vena cava, or the portal vein. An atrial septal defect is essential for survival. The hemodynamics are similar to those of a large atrial septal defect.

aortic stenosis (AS) Obstruction to LV outflow. This may occur at valvular, supravalvular, or subvalvular levels. The subvalvular obstruction may occasionally be due to a congenital fibrous ring just below the aortic valve (discrete subvalvular AS), but usually it is due to a hypertrophied septum impinging on the anterior leaflet of the mitral valve during systole (hypertrophic subaortic stenosis, hypertrophic obstructive cardiomyopathy). (See figure, p. 203.) The supravalvular type is associated with a characteristic facies (see p. 21). Aortic valvular stenosis without any other valves involved is almost always congenital, and about half of these are due to calcification of a bicuspid aortic valve. The acquired ones are usually due to rheumatic valvulitis and are associated with some mitral valve disease. In subjects over age 70, degenerative calcification of the aortic valve may be the most common cause of aortic stenosis, especially in women.

arteriosclerosis 1. Atherosclerosis (the progressive laying down of lipid in the intima of an artery, starting with a fatty streak and ending with a plaque made up of lipids, fibrosis, and calcium). 2. Medial sclerosis (fibrosis of the media or muscular layers of arteries, which may end in "pipestem" arteries). Medial sclerosis affects only the larger peripheral arteries; i.e., the aorta and coronary arteries are subject to atherosclerosis but not to medial sclerosis. Arterioles are not usually affected either by medial sclerosis or atherosclerosis.

atrial myxoma A tumor made up of soft, loose, friable tissue that is usually on a pedicle (pendunculated) attached to the atrial septum in the region of the fossa ovalis. It is almost twice as common in the left atrium as in the right atrium. It can protrude through its respective atrioventricular (AV) valve in diastole to produce a partial obstruction that imitates mitral or tricuspid stenosis and occasionally causes syncope. It may merely prevent complete closure of the valve, resulting in various degrees of mitral or tricuspid regurgitation. If the tumor becomes calcified, it may act like a wrecking ball and completely destroy the AV valve, producing severe regurgitation. Emboli from the friable tumor are among the most common causes of clinical manifestations. For unknown reasons, the tumor acts as an inflammatory agent and commonly produces a high sedimentation rate and intermittent fevers, which, together with the occasional clubbing, mimics infective endocarditis. It may even produce reactions of an allergic type, resulting in puzzling skin and joint manifestations.

atrial septal defect (ASD) An opening between the atria, which may occur at three possible levels. The lower one is called a *primum defect*, the middle one is a *secundum defect*, and the upper one is called a *sinus venosus defect*. By far the most common is the secundum, or fossa ovalis defect.

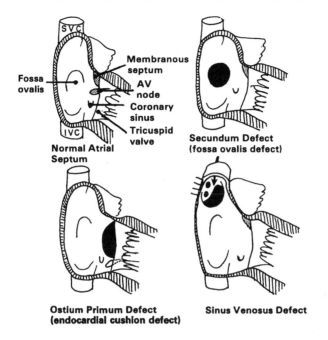

The three levels of atrial septal defects are, in general, low, middle, and high. It may help your memory if you think of the lower two levels as the "first floor," or primum defect, and the "second floor," or secundum defect. The sinus venosus defect then remains and thus must be the "top floor," or high defect. The sinus venosus is the embryological site of the pacemaker of the heart, or the sinoatrial node. If you keep in mind that the sino-atrial node is at the junction of the superior vena cava and right atrium, it will be easy to remember that the sinus venosus defect is the high one. When the inferior wall of the fossa ovalis acts like a flap valve, it is called a patent foremen ovale. There will then be flow from the right to the left atrium only if the pressure rises abnormally high in the right atrium. The flap is normally closed by the higher pressure in the left atrium relative to that in the right atrium. Note that in the sinus venosus defect, two anomalous pulmonary veins are shown draining info the superior vena cava.

primum defect An atrial septal defect that is part of a possible spectrum of abnormalities caused by maldevelopment of the fetal heart that give rise to

1. The inferior part of the atrial septum above.
2. The upper part of the ventricular septum below.

3. The medial (anterior) leaflet of the mitral valve on the left.
4. The septal leaflet of the tricuspid valve on the right.

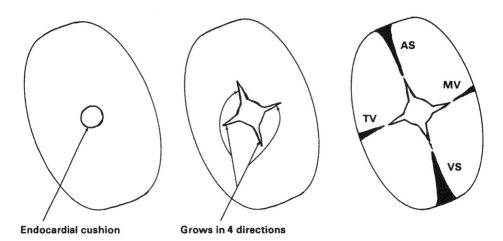

Endocardial cushion   **Grows in 4 directions**

If the lower part of the atrial septum (AS) does not develop, an ostium primum ASD results. If the upper part of the ventricular septum (VS) is missing, a ventricular septal defect results. If the medial cushion parts of the mitral (MV) or tricuspid valves (TV) are missing, a cleft mitral or tricuspid leaflet results.

Any permutation or combination of endocardial cushion defects may occur. When defects in all four of the above structures are present, the condition is called a *complete atrioventricular canal* or complete endocardial cushion defect. A left axis deviation on ECG is so common with endocardial cushion defects and so rare with atrial septal defects at higher levels that for the clinical differentiation of the primum from the secundum and sinus venosus defects by ECG it is quite helpful.

sinus venosus defect A high atrial septal defect that is always associated with an anomalous drainage of one or two right pulmonary veins into the superior vena cava. (See **anomalous pulmonary venous connection or drainage**.)

The shunted blood in atrial septal defects travels from the left to the right atrium, from the right atrium to the right ventricle, from the right ventricle to the pulmonary artery, from the pulmonary artery to the pulmonary arterioles and veins, and from the pulmonary veins to the left atrium. Therefore, the right atrium, right ventricle, and pulmonary vessels all have a volume overload. The left atrium, however, serves only as a conduit and does not become enlarged except under exceptional circumstances. (See figure on p. 271.)

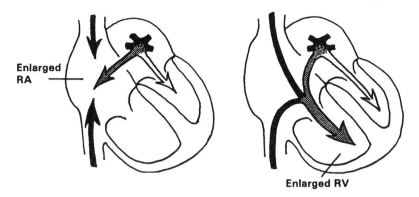

Note that with an atrial septal defect, the right atrium and ventricle receive blood from two sources. They are volume-overloaded at the expense of blood to the left ventricle. An increase in total blood volume is the compensatory mechanism by which the left ventricle receives a normal volume for average physiological needs. When an atrial septal defect or any other left-to-right shunt is closed surgically, the total blood volume of the body decreases by the exact amount of the shunt.

atrioventricular block (AV block) Conduction delay anywhere from the AV node to the ending of the bundle branches in the ventricle, i.e., the delay may occur in the AV node, the bundle of His, or the bundle branches. A first-degree AV block is recognized by seeing a long P–R interval. Second-degree AV block refers to intermittent complete AV block in which a dropped QRS occurs periodically. If the AV block is complete, the atria and ventricles are dissociated and an independent pacemaker for the ventricles occurs either at or below the bundle of His.

atrioventricular dissociation A condition in which the atria and ventricles have independent pacemakers. The lower pacemaker may be in the junctional area or deep in a ventricle. AV dissociation implies that atrial contraction has varying relationships to ventricular contraction, i.e., if the atria are in sinus rhythm, the P–R interval will be continually changing in a haphazard manner.

beriberi heart disease The effect on the heart of total body capillary dilatation caused by a deficiency of vitamin B_1 (thiamine). In order to fill the enlarged vascular bed, a marked hypervolemic, hyperkinetic state is produced, with a high venous pressure, tachycardia, cardiomegaly, peripheral edema, and rapid circulation time. In the occident, it is seen almost entirely in alcoholic persons who resort to an enormous intake of beer. An acute, fulminant, nonedematous form characterized by cardiovascular collapse and death within hours or days has been called *shoshin beriberi*. (*Sho* is Japanese for "damage," and *shin* means "heart").

Bernoulli effect The drop in pressure on the surface of any structure caused by a flow over that structure. This tends to pull the structure toward the stream. An instrument utilizing the Bernoulli effect to measure flow is called a Venturi meter. The Bernoulli effect on the wings of an airplane raises it and keeps it airborne.

carcinoid heart disease Accumulation of grossly whitish yellow fibrous tissue on the inner surface of the right ventricle or atrium, as well as on the undersurface of the tricuspid and pulmonary valves (rarely, of the mitral valve). It can hold the tricuspid or pulmonary valve in the semiclosed position and so cause tricuspid or pulmonary stenosis and regurgitation. Carcinoid heart disease is usually associated with a carcinoid tumor of the bowel and with metastases to the liver. Bronchospasm, diarrhea, and various types of flushing (general redness, bright red patches, or violaceous cyanosis) are all part of the carcinoid syndrome.

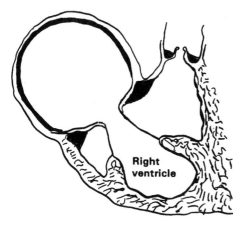

Carcinoid deposits tend to form on the undersurface of the tricuspid valves and the upper surface of the pulmonary valves and so hold them in a rigid, semiclosed position. The compliance of the right atrium can be reduced by a lining of carcinoid material, thus raising its pressure conspicuously.

cardiomyopathy Myocardial damage from any cause. Therefore, it should have an adjective preceding it, e.g., idiopathic cardiomyopathy (often called primary myocardial disease or dilated cardiomyopathy), amyloid cardiomyopathy, or coronary or ischemic cardiomyopathy.

Cheyne-Stokes respiration The periodic breathing characterized by a gradually increasing depth of respiration, culminating in a period of apena that may last from a few seconds to as long as a minute. During the period of apnea, the oxygen saturation reaches its lowest level and the carbon dioxide tension its highest, causing the cycle to be repeated again. The most common associated condition for the cardiologist is severe low output due to heart failure. The neurologist more commonly sees it as a result of cerebral disease. Because it is exaggerated when dozing, and the hyperpneic phase can cause enough cerebral stimulation to prevent sleep, it is a possible cause of insomnia in a patient with heart failure.

circulation time The time it takes for a marker material to travel from the site of injection to the site of appearance, usually after it passes through the lungs or lesser circulation.

clubbing A condition in which soft tissue of the terminal phalanges of the fingers or toes becomes hypertrophied and the nail finally curves excessively, giving a drumstick appearance. (See p. 17 for method of eliciting.) In cardiac patients, clubbing is usually associated with cyanosis, but if not, it should suggest the presence of acute infective endocarditis that has been present for a few weeks, suppurative lung lesions, anoxic cor pulmonale, or metastatic lung cancer. More rarely, it is caused by chronic diarrhea with ulcerative colitis or may even be familial. In cardiac patients, the most common causes of clubbing are tetralogy of Fallot and transposition of the great vessels. When clubbing and cyanosis are greater in the toes than in the hands, the condition is called differential cyanosis (see p. 237) and clubbing. (See illustrations at beginning of Chapter 2, Questions 3 and 4.)

coarctation Localized or diffuse narrowing of the aorta. The degree of constriction varies from slight to severe; rarely, it is complete. It is usually seen around the isthmus, which is the area just beyond both the left subclavian artery and the ductus arteriosus. It can occur proximal to the left subclavian artery and occasionally even in the abdominal aorta. Collateral vessels develop through the internal mammary and shoulder girdle arteries to the intercostal arteries and can become very large and even palpable. In all the vessels proximal to the coarctation, there is hypertension and increased pulse pressure as well as dilatation. There is a very low systolic pressure and pulse pressure beyond the coarctation.

The aortic valve is commonly bicuspid and regurgitant, but is occasionally stenotic.

Preductal coarctation is commonly associated with diffuse narrowing of the aortic arch, pulmonary hypertension, and an Eisenmenger syndrome, as well as with differential cyanosis (see p. 18). This is sometimes known as the infantile type, because patients rarely live beyond infancy.

compliance Elastic resistance or stiffness of a structure, e.g., the stiffer the left ventricle, the less the compliance. To physicists it is change of volume/change of pressure. Generally, a thick ventricle is a noncompliant or stiff ventricle.

constrictive pericarditis Thickening of the pericardium by dense, fibrous tissue that may calcify. It results primarily in restriction of expansion of the heart but also often causes a slight restriction of systole as well, especially if the duration of the constriction is long enough to allow much infiltration of the epicardium by the fibrous tissue. In past decades the most common cause was tuberculosis. The most common causes today are idiopathic, viral, bacterial, radiotherapy of the chest, and hemopericardium resulting from trauma.

Restrictive cardiomyopathy mimics constrictive pericarditis, but restrictive disease is more likely to have cardiomegaly (displaced apex beat), and its S_3 is more likely loudest at the apex. In constriction the S_3 may be loudest at the left lower sternal border.

cor pulmonale Right ventricular hypertrophy secondary to a lung abnormality, such as primary pulmonary hypertension. The term does not require that the patient be in right ventricular failure.

ductus arteriosus See **persistent ductus arteriosus**.

Ebstein's anomaly A downward-displaced, deformed tricuspid valve. One leaflet is displaced into the right ventricle (RV) so that some RV is in the right atrium. There is commonly tricuspid regurgitation, which can enlarge the outflow tract of the RV. The right atrium may be so large that it dominates the ECG (tall peaked P waves) and X-ray picture. A right-to-left shunt through an atrial septal defect or patent foremen ovale with resultant cyanosis is common. Atrial arrythmias or heart failure are the most common complications.

Eisenmenger syndrome or reaction Severe pulmonary hypertension due to high and fixed pulmonary arteriolar resistance caused by a large left-to-right shunt due to a ventricular septal defect (VSD), atrial septal defect (ASD), or persistent ductus arteriosus (PDA). The high right ventricular and right atrial pressures result in a right-to-left shunt through the ASD, VSD, or PDA. The right-to-left shunt may be dominant or it may be a balanced shunt, i.e., as much left-to-right as right-to-left. When a VSD is the cause, the term *Eisenmenger complex* is often used, because this is the original lesion described by Eisenmenger in 1897 [1]. The Eisenmenger syndrome usually begins in infancy when a PDA or VSD is responsible; it begins in the teens or later when the shunt is an ASD. The pulmonary hypertension of Eisenmenger syndrome with cyanosis is irreversible and prohibits surgical closure of the defect. A patient with irreversible pathological changes in the lung vessels (plexiform lesions) due to an Eisenmenger reaction is often said to have "pulmonary vascular disease."

ejection fraction Relationship between stroke volume (volume ejected) and end-diastolic volume (volume at the moment of greatest filling of the ventricle at the end of diastole). It is the volume at the end of diastole minus the volume at the end of systole divided by the volume at the end of diastole, times 100. (The normal range is $70 \pm 10\%$.)

endocardial cushion defect See **atrial septal defect**.

endocarditis See **infective endocarditis**.

Fallot's tetralogy See **tetralogy of Fallot**.

filling pressure The pressure in the ventricle that distends it, especially toward the end of diastole, so that it is most related to the end-diastolic pressure in the ventricle. The change in volume that produces this diastolic pressure is called the preload. It is controlled on the right side by venous pressure and, in sinus rhythm, also by the power of the right atrial contraction. On the left side it is controlled by the left atrial pressure and, in sinus rhythm, also by the power of left atrial contraction or the "atrial kick."

gradient Difference in pressure along a conduit that results in flow from highest to lowest pressure. In cardiology, it usually refers to a difference in pressure across an obstruction, i.e., it is generally caused by a drop in pressure across an obstruction (usually a stenotic artery or valve), so that the pressure is higher proximal than distal to the obstruction.

hypertelorism Widely set eyes found in such syndromes as pulmonary stenosis with atrial septal defect and with supravalvular aortic stenosis.

hypertrophic obstructive cardiomyopathy Disproportionate hypertrophy of the septum that causes obstruction in midsystole as the anterior or septal mitral leaflet draws toward the septum in systole. (See figures on p. 203 for hemodynamics). The disproportionate septal hypertrophy has engendered the term *asymmetric septal hypertrophy*. It was called idiopathic hypertrophic subaortic stenosis in the first extensive report, but the term *idiopathic* seems an unnecessary appendage [2]. *Asymmetric septal hypertrophy* (commonly called ASH) does not necessarily imply obstruction to outflow, since ASH can occur without obstruction. Therefore, *hypertrophic obstructive cardiomyopathy* (HOCM) should be used when referring to a patient with obstruction due to asymmetric septal hypertrophy.

infective endocarditis An infection usually of regurgitant heart valves or of certain congenital defects that cause regurgitant or retrograde flows, such as ventricular septal defect or persistent ductus arteriosus. In former years, the infection was nearly always bacterial and thus the condition was called bacterial endocarditis. Because it could last for as long as 2 years before the diagnosis was made, it was known as subacute bacterial endocarditis. Today, fungi and *Rickettsia* are the causative organisms in a significant proportion of infections. Therefore, *infective* is a more embracing term.

The diagnosis used to be considered when there was fever and "changing murmurs." Because a regurgitant murmur is the only murmur likely to develop when a valve is destroyed, the term *changing* should be modified to mean a new or increasing *regurgitant* valvular murmur. Patients often have had recent dental work or other surgery and may present with severe night sweats, back pain, cerebral vascular accident, or other embolic phenomena.

inflow and outflow tract of the left ventricle The inflow tract of the left ventricle is the area just below the mitral valve. The outflow tract is made up of the septum anteromedially and the anterior or septal leaflet of the mitral valve, plus their chordae laterally. (See figure on p. 207.)

infundibulum Outflow tract of the right ventricle made up mostly of muscle called the crista supraventricularis. It is much like the spout of a teapot, the body of the right ventricle being the pot. (See figure on p. 207.)

intermittent claudication Pain in ischemic working muscle produced by certain metabolites; classically, pain in the legs due to inadequate arterial supply during walking. If the obstruction is high in the aortoiliac area, the pain may be in the hip or buttock. However, the pain may be felt in unusual sites, such as in the thighs or the arch of the foot. When the ischemia is due to thrombosis of the lower aorta (chronic aortoiliac occlusion), impotence and leg weakness may occur as well (Leriche's syndrome) [3]. If the celiac or mesenteric arteries are involved, the pain after meals is called "abdominal angina."

Note: Intermittent claudication is not related to the nocturnal leg or foot muscle cramps that occur in bed.

ischemia (pronounced **is-ke-mi-ah**) Inadequate blood supply to a part of the body.

isovolumic contraction The rise in LV pressure between closure of the mitral valve and opening of the aortic valve. This used to be called isometric contraction, but because the measurements of the ventricle change while the volume does not, the term *isovolumic* is more accurate.

isovolumic relaxation The fall in LV pressure between closure of the aortic valve and opening of the mitral valve.

Note: Isovolumic relaxation is an active process, i.e., the ventricle is capable of generating a negative pressure or suction" effect.

left lateral decubitus position Body position in which the subject is horizontal and lying on the left side.

malpositions of the heart *Situs solitus* (*solitus* = "usual") means a normal position of all chambers and vessels of the heart and viscera. In *situs inversus* or mirror-image dextrocardia all chambers, vessels, and viscera are inverted with the apex, etc. on the right. Dextrocardia or levocardia means that the heart and viscera are discordant and are almost always associated with other cardiac abnormalities. Dextroversion or levoversion means that the heart is in the same position as in dextrocardia or levocardia but the heart is rotated so that the apex is rotated to the left with dextroversion and to the right with levoversion.

Marfan syndrome See index for clinical descriptions in text.

medial sclerosis See **arteriosclerosis**.

Mueller maneuver An inspiratory effort against a closed mouth and nose or against a closed glottis that decreases intrathoracic pressure. It is the opposite of a **Valsalva maneuver**.

neurocirculatory asthenia A syndrome occurring in some patients with anxiety neurosis and consisting of palpitations and tachycardias, nondescript chest pains, shortness of breath, chronic fatigue, and other signs of sympathetic overactivity. It has been called DaCosta's syndrome (American Civil War), "soldier's heart" (World War II), "effort syndrome," "neurotic heart syndrome," "cardiac neurosis," and "vasoregulatory asthenia." If these patients are chronic hyperventilators, their breath-holding time will be less than 20 s.

outflow tract See **inflow and outflow tract of the left ventricle**.

patent ductus arteriosus See **persistent ductus arteriosus**.

pectus excavatum Posterior displacement of the lower sternum. It can be slight, or so severe that it not only displaces the heart to the left but also may interfere with cardiac function by raising the right ventricular diastolic pressure and may cause palpitations and dyspnea on strenuous exertions. It is commonly seen in the **Marfan syndrome** and in patients with the straight back syndrome (see p. 196). The three degrees of severity have been described as the "saucer," "cup," and "funnel."

persistent ductus arteriosus (PDA) Usually incorrectly called patent ductus arteriosus. The word *ductus* itself implies patency [4]. It refers to an opening between the aorta and pulmonary artery in which flow occurs between the higher-pressure aorta and the lower-pressure pulmonary artery. Thus some of the blood ejected by the LV into the aorta passes into the pulmonary artery, resulting in a left-to-right shunt. A volume overload occurs where the shunted blood circulates, i.e., in the pulmonary artery, pulmonary veins, left atrium, and LV. In uncomplicated PDA, the right-sided chambers should be normal.

A PDA represents persistence of the fetal ductus arteriosus that is designed to bypass the lungs in fetal life, i.e., the high pulmonary artery pressure in the fetus forces blood into the aorta through the ductus. In PDA severe pulmonary hypertension may develop if the fetal arterioles do not involute. When pulmonary hypertension develops, its onset usually occurs early in infancy or childhood. Then the right ventricle remains hypertrophied, resulting in an Eisenmenger syndrome or reaction with right-to-left shunting. If a patient with a large PDA reaches adulthood without developing pulmonary hypertension in infancy, heart failure with acute pulmonary edema may develop. Infective endocarditis can occur as one of the complications of even a small PDA. (See p. 237 under PDA for an explanation of differential cyanosis, which is one of the characteristics of the Eisenmenger reaction in persistent ductus arteriosus.)

postextrasystolic potentiation Increased contractility that occurs in the beat following a premature electrical depolarization of the heart. Although a pause after a premature beat can increase contractility by the long diastole, causing more fill-

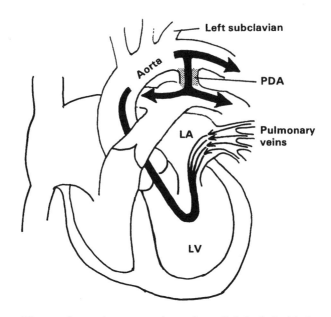

The persistent ductus arteriosus is a slightly left-sided structure that usually connects the junction of the main and pulmonary artery to the aorta just distal to the origin of the left subclavian artery. Since normal aortic pressure (120/80 mmHg) is usually higher than pulmonary artery pressure (25/10 mmHg), the shunt flow is normally from aorta to pulmonary artery in both systole and diastole.

ing and a Starling effect, an early depolarization itself produces increased contractility, i.e., contractility that is independent of the length of diastole following the early beat. The cause of this increased inotropism is thought to be a calcium flux phenomenon.

postmyocardial infarction syndrome (Dressler's syndrome [5]) A syndrome consisting of fever, pneumonitis, and painful pericarditis and pleuritis that may occur from about 2 to 11 weeks after myocardial infarction and is probably an autoimmune response to myocardial necrosis. It is only dangerous in the presence of anticoagulants, when it may produce a bloody effusion and tamponade. The syndrome closely resembles the postcardiotomy syndrome and may be recurrent for as long as 2 years.

primary pulmonary hypertension Irreversible pulmonary hypertension of unknown etiology, usually progressing to severe degrees, producing right ventricular hypertrophy and dilatation, as well as main pulmonary artery dilatation and atherosclerosis. It is most common in females under age 40. The small pulmonary arteries and arterioles show intimal fibrosis and proliferation as well as medial thickening.

pulse pressure or volume Amplitude of a pulse. In palpation, it refers to the distance your fingers are moved between the least and the greatest expansion of a vessel. On an arterial pulse tracing, it refers to the distance between the systolic and diastolic pressures.

Raynaud's phenomenon Intermittent constriction of small arteries and arterioles of the fingers, resulting in a change of color, usually produced by cooling but also by sympathetic stimulation of any kind. It begins with blanching, progresses to cyanosis, and often ends with a reactive redness (reactive hyperemia) that may be very painful. It is occasionally a precursor of a collagen or other connective-tissue disease. It is called Raynaud's *disease* when it is not secondary to trauma or to neurogenic lesions or other systemic disease.

Note: Acrocyanosis is a persistent blueness and coldness of the distal parts of the extremities, probably due to an abnormality of the small vessels.

semilunar valves The aortic or pulmonary valves. Their leaflets are half-moon-shaped (semilunar).

sinus arrhythmia Increase in heart rate with inspiration and decrease with expiration due to vagal inhibition during inspiration. (Remember "in" for "increase" on inspiration.)

sinuses of Valsalva The three bulges or sinuses at the root of the aorta, two of which give rise to the coronary arteries. They help to prevent the open aortic leaflets from occluding the orifice of the coronary arteries. Occasionally, they may be congenitally weak and rupture into adjacent chambers, or they may become aneurysmal, especially in the Marfan syndrome, producing any degree of aortic regurgitation. (See top figure on p. 280.)

Starling effect The effect of the Frank-Starling law of the heart, which states that if the heart muscle is stretched before it contracts, it will contract with more energy. This is equivalent to a bow-and-arrow effect, i.e., the tauter the bow, the farther the arrow will go.

sternal angle, or angle of Louis (pronounced **Loo-ee**) The first protuberance or hump in the sternum below the suprasternal notch. It is at the junction of the manubrium and body of the sternum. It marks the point where the second costal cartilage joins the sternum. Below this cartilage is the second intercostal space. (See bottom figure on p. 280.)

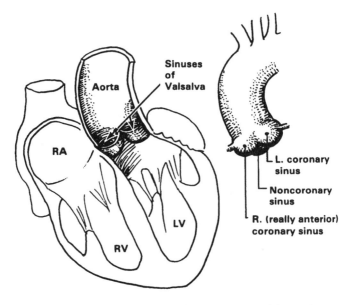

The right coronary sinus is anterior when viewed from above, but it is called the right coronary sinus, probably because it gives rise to the right coronary artery.

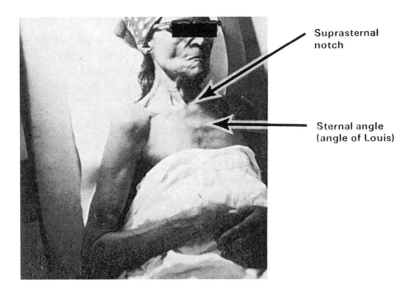

The sternal angle is one of the most important landmarks in cardiology, not only because it is the zero level for jugular pressures but also because it is the only accurate way to find the fourth right interspace in order to place the V_1 electrode for an ECG.

Stokes-Adams attack or Adams-Stokes attack An episode of syncope secondary to complete AV block (see **atrioventricular block**). Any cerebral symptom secondary to complete AV block may probably also be considered a minor degree of Stokes-Adams attack because it may presage syncope and death. Syncope secondary to any other arrhythmia should probably be called cardiac syncope and not a Stokes-Adams attack.

subclavian steal Use of a vertebral artery as collateral circulation to feed a subclavian artery beyond an obstruction (usually on the left). Blood from a vertebral artery flows retrogradely into the distal subclavian, thus "stealing" blood from the brain.

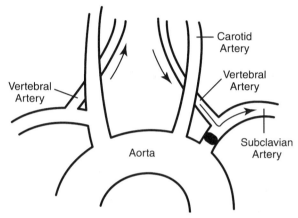

If the left subclavian is blocked proximal to the entrance of the left vertebral artery, exercise of the ischemic left arm causes blood in the right vertebral artery to flow via intracerebral vessels into the left vertebral, which then flows retrogradely downward into the subclavian beyond the obstruction. The blood drawn from the cerebral circulation causes cerebral ischemia with resultant vertigo, ataxia, or dysarthria.

tamponade Restriction of cardiac diastole caused by fluid in the pericardium. Because the pressure in the pericardium is equal to venous pressure, the patient with tamponade must of necessity have a high venous pressure and usually also have peripheral edema when the tamponade becomes severe. Pericardial effusion without a high venous pressure is not tamponade. A combination of fluid and solid pericardial material causing constriction is called *effusive-constrictive pericarditis*. A useful method of detecting pericardial fluid is to listen to the heart sounds and murmurs first lying supine, then while the patient is on his or her stomach and propped up on the elbows. If there is fluid gravitating anteriorly, the sounds become softer, instead of louder as in normal subjects.

tetralogy of Fallot The most common congenital heart abnormality, it refers to a large ventricular septal defect, pulmonary stenosis, an overriding aorta, and right ventricular hypertrophy (RVH). Because pulmonary stenosis will always lead to RVH, the latter is a necessary result of the other congenital lesions and not really part of the basic abnormality.

The pulmonary stenosis may be either valvular, infundibular, or both, and is the cause of the murmur. The enlargement of the aorta by virtue of receiving blood from both ventricles may contribute to the overriding.

A right aortic arch is relatively frequent. Its pulsation should be sought just below the right sternoclavicular joint, which itself may be felt to pulsate.

thrill A vibratory sensation similar to what is felt when touching the head and neck of a purring cat. A long thrill is merely a palpable murmur and signifies that the murmur is at least grade 4/6 in loudness. A short thrill on the chest wall may be a juxtaposition of split heart sound vibrations. A short thrill felt on the carotid artery may be due to a mid-systolic dip or a minor degree of bisferiens pulse.

transposition of the great vessels It is often called "complete" transposition of the great vessels and means that the anteroposterior relationship of the aorta and pulmonary arteries is reversed, i.e., instead of the aortic root being posterior to the pulmonary artery, it is anterior (and often to the right). This results in the right ventricle giving rise to the aorta and the left ventricle giving rise to the pulmonary artery. One or more abnormal communications between the systemic and pulmonary circulation must exist for the patient to survive. Mixing may occur through either an atrial septal defect, a ventricular septal defect, a persistent ductus, or large bronchial arteries.

Cyanosis is usually present either from birth or within a few days of birth. The most common cause of cyanosis combined with shunt vascularity in the lungs on X-ray is transposition of the great vessels, especially if it is accompanied by congestive failure in infancy.

Turner's syndrome Female phenotype consisting of short stature, receding chin, webbed neck, low hairline over the back of the neck, broad shield chest resulting in widely separated nipples, exaggerated carrying angle, sparse axillary and pubic hair, lymphedema of the lower extremities (in infancy), and a short fourth metacarpal. It is sometimes simply described as short stature, neck webbing, and sexual infantilism in a female with a sex chromosome abnormality (absence of one of the two sex chromosomes). Coarctation of the aorta is the most common associated cardiovascular lesion. When patients with such an appearance have normal sex chromosomes and also have hypertelorism with a slight antimongoloid slant to the eyes as well as ptosis of the upper lids and exophthalmos, especially if the above physical characteristics are found in a male, they are likely to have pulmonary stenosis and are said to have Noonan's syndrome.

Valsalva maneuver (See also the section on blood pressure response on pp. 59–61.) A forced expiration against a closed glottis in order to raise intrathoracic pressure. There are several methods for helping patients perform this maneuver. (1) Have patient blow into an anaeroid manometer until it registers 40 mmHg. (2) Have patient push his or her abdomen against your hand. (3) Have patient seal his or her lips around his index finger and blow hard on the finger for about 10 s.

The rise in intrathoracic pressure (phase 1) decreases venous return to the heart, thus causing a gradual decrease in heart size, stroke volume, and pulse pressure. There is a tachycardia due to reflex sympathetic stimulation as the blood pressure falls (phase 2). On release of the strain there is a further sudden drop of blood pressure for a few beats because of the almost empty pulmonary venous reservoir (phase 3). The blood that had been dammed up in the venae cavae now pours into the lungs, LV, and aorta. The heart rate now slows and an excessive rise in blood pressure occurs for a few beats due to the reflex sympathetic stimulation caused by the strain that takes a few seconds to be "turned off," plus the effect of the sudden increase in volume distending the carotid baroreceptors.

ventricular aneurysm See **aneurysm**.

ventricular septal defect An opening or hole in the ventricular septum is the most common congenital lesion. It is most usually found in the translucent membranous portion of the ventricle, a few centimeters below the aortic valve. It may, however, be found in the muscular septum, in the supracristal area leading directly into the pulmonary artery (rare), or posterior and superior to the attachment of the tricuspid valve to the membranous septum and therefore may lead directly into the right atrium (Gerbode defect). Ventricular septal defect shunts occur mostly during systole from left to right, i.e., from the left to the right ventricle, and produce volume overloads in the right ventricle, pulmonary artery, pulmonary veins, left atrium, and left ventricle.

The defect varies in size from pinpoint to slightly more than a centimeter in diameter. When it involves the entire septum, a single ventricle is produced. When multiple muscular defects are present, it is known as a *Swiss cheese defect*. Unless the defect is very large, the hole may close in the first few years of life, often with a membranous septal pouch or aneurysm. (See figure on p. 284.)

A dreaded complication of large defects is severe pulmonary hypertension, which may become irreversible. When it becomes severe enough to reverse the shunt, this is known as an Eisenmenger complex (see **Eisenmenger syndrome**), and usually occurs within the first years of life.

Wolff-Parkinson-White (W-P-W) preexcitation This refers to an atrioventricular bypass pathway in which an abnormal conduction pathway between the atrium and ventricle bypasses the AV node, thus shortening the P–R interval and producing a wide QRS.

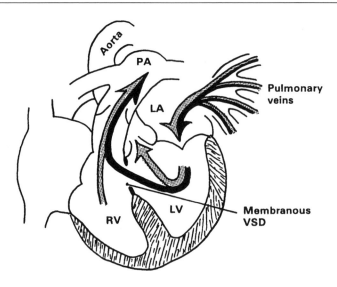

In most ventricular septal defects, only the right atrium is
spared the volume overload caused by the left-to-right shunt.
In the rare left ventricle-to-right atrium type of ventricular
septal defect, however, all cardiac chambers are volume-overloaded. In this figure, the black portion of the arrow represents the shunt flow, and the dotted portion represents the
normal flow that comes from the venae cavae.

xanthoma A cholesterol-filled nodule found either subcutaneously or over a tendon.
Tuberous xanthomas are subcutaneous xanthomas on the extensor surfaces of the
extremities. They are associated with an increase in coronary disease and high
blood levels of both cholesterol and triglycerides. They are most commonly found
in patients with type III (high-IDL) hyperlipoproteinemia but also with type II
(high cholesterol) or type IV (high triglycerides). Since they are under the skin,
their yellow pigment is visible. Tendon xanthomas are too deep to impart any
change of color to the skin.

  eruptive xanthomas Tiny yellowish nodules 1–2 cm in diameter on an erythema-
  tous base and found mostly on pressure areas. They are often transient and
  vary with the degree of hypertriglyceridemia, with which they are associated.
  The triglyceride level is usually at least 1000 mg per 100 mL, no matter what
  the cause, whether diabetes or pure type I hyperlipoproteinomia. There is some
  correlation with coronary disease.

  palmer xanthomas Very small xanthomas found in the palmer crease and probably representing an early stage of the tuberous type.

REFERENCES

1. Eisenmenger, F. Die angeborenen Defect de Kammerscheidewand de Herzens. *Stschr. Klin. Med.* 32:1, 1897.
2. Braunwald, E., et al. Idiopathic hypertrophic subaortic stenosis: Description based on analysis of 64 patients. *Circulation* 29 (Suppl. 14):1, 1964.
3. Leriche, R., and Morel, A. The syndrome of thrombotic obliteration of the aortic bifurcation. *Ann. Surg.* 127:193, 1958.
4. Marguis, R. M., and Godman, M. J. Nomenclature of the ductus arteriosus. *Br. Heart J.* 49:288, 1983.
5. Dressler, W. The post-myocardial infarction syndrome. *Arch. Intern. Med.* 103: 28, 1959.

Index

About the Author

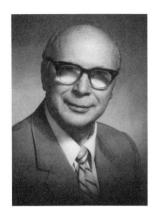

Jules Constant, MD, FACC, graduated from the University of Toronto, and is a Clinical Associate Professor of Medicine at the State University of New York at Buffalo.

He is the author of *Learning Electrocardiography, A Complete Course (4th Edition), Essentials of Learning Electrocardiography for Students and Housestaff,* and *Six Cassettes of a Complete Course in Auscultation,* and numerous articles on clinical cardiology.

He has lectured as Annual Visiting Professor for two months a year in Japanese hospitals for 29 years (over 75 hospitals), and in Taiwan and Philippine hospitals for two weeks annually for 15 years.

A Complete Course in Heart Sounds and Murmurs on CD

PRODUCED BY
Jules Constant, MD, FACC, and Tom Greene
Produced at Grenadier in Rochester, NY
GA7021

The audio CD attached to the back cover is playable in any standard audio device, including computers equipped with sound card and speakers. For optimal results, headphones with good bass response should be used.

DISK INDICES:

1	Introduction	(00:16)	11	HOCM	(04:00)	
2	S_1 Splitting	(11:42)	12	Mitral Regurgitation	(07:28)	
3	S_2 Splitting	(05:52)	13	Mitral Valve Prolapse	(04:36)	
4	Opening Snap	(04:33)	14	VSD	(01:09)	
5	S_3	(05:29)	15	Mitral Stenosis	(02:56)	
6	Atrial Myxoma	(01:22)	16	Aortic Regurgitation	(02:49)	
7	S_4	(02:48)	17	Austin Flint Murmur	(02:08)	
8	Double Gallop	(01:08)	18	PDA	(01:51)	
9	Ejection Murmurs	(06:32)	19	Venous Hum	(01:51)	
10	Still's Murmur	(02:15)	20	Friction Rubs	(01:10)	
			21	Beethoven's Opening Snap	(01:48)	

Limited Warranty and Disclaimer